THE
REVENGE
DIET

Also by Monica Grenfell

Fabulous in a Fortnight

Monica's Fabulous Body Plan: Fantastic Legs & Thighs

Monica's Fabulous Body Plan: Best Bust, Arms and Back

Monica's Fabulous Body Plan:Marvelllous Midriff

Monica's Fabulous Body Plan:Beautiful Bottom

Beat Your Body Chaos

Cellulite Buster: the 30-Day Diet

The New Get Back Into Your Jeans Diet

The New 5 Days To A Flatter Stomach

Monica GRENFELL

THE REVENGE DIET

Make him sorry he dumped you!
— Lose 15lbs in a month

MONTGOMERY

First published in Great Britain in 2007 by
Montgomery Books
P.O Box 64
Oxfordshire
Ox12 9GA

www.monicagrenfell.co.uk

ISBN 978 0952 600411

10 9 8 7 6 5 4 3 2 1

A CIP catalogue record for this book is available from
the British Library.

Printed and bound in Great Britain by Booksprint,
Wellington, Somerset.

Contents

Acknowledgements

Abby, Abi, Caroline, Celia, Christina, Helen, Lilli, Liz,
Michelle, Nicola, Sadie, Sue.

Visit Monica's website at
www.monicagrenfell.co.uk

FOREWORD

I had been dumped by the love of my life only two weeks before; left on a park bench, crying pitifully. I had not planned to meet him that day, but we bumped into each other by chance, me slightly embarrassed because he had caught me with flyaway hair, no make-up and badly-fitting jeans and him looking quite the opposite: meltingly gorgeous, unusually well-groomed. He suggested we have a walk. I started talking plans for next week, next month. He looked at the ground and took a deep breath. Then he finished with me.

We'd had a blistering affair. We couldn't imagine being apart; we were truly, madly, deeply in love. I burned with lust when I was with him and pined with pain and longing when we were apart. I could hardly do a day's work for thinking about him. He told me he felt the same. I wanted to be with him for the rest of my life and he wanted me. At least that's how it had been. But something happened at New Year and here he was, January 6th and it was all over.

I didn't figure in his plans, he said. He was sorry, but he'd met somebody else. She was waiting in his car, actually, and (here he glanced at his watch) would I mind awfully if he went because she would wonder where he was?

That was it. Boom. And he was walking away and I would never see him again. I was finished.

Actually I did see him again. Two weeks later, ten pounds thinner and deeply depressed, I walked out of the hairdresser and there he was. I had been wandering round town early one morning wondering what to do with myself and can you believe I went to get my hair done and met him?

Monica GRENFELL

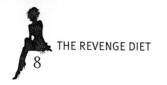
What unbelievable luck. "Monica" he said. He shook his head and blew out his cheeks. "you —er- look fantastic".

It wasn't world-class. But it was something. I told that tale for years to all my girlfriends who felt similarly let down, broken hearted or dumped. "Go and have your hair done" I would say, "Or at least get it washed. Put on something sexy. If you can't eat and the weight's falling off, well, every cloud has a silver lining. Get what you can out of this. And who knows, if you bump into him, at least you'll be looking fantastic and he might just be sorry. And if he isn't sorry, at least he'll remember how great you looked"

Incidentally, it would be twenty-three years until I saw him again. I'll tell you later.

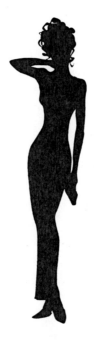

Monica GRENFELL

INTRODUCTION

True Stories

Anne's story

I thought I'd never get over my broken heart. I was nobody's endless victim, but it hurt all the same. I had nobody to get revenge on except him. He'd found somebody else but had worked us in tandem until she was truly up and running and he could afford to cut me adrift, like a glider that has been hauled to the heights where it can catch the air currents and go it alone. But in fairness, he hadn't done anything wrong. Relationships end. We weren't married. I could hardly blame him for something I had done myself, to other people. Ending a relationship is normal but how you react can be anything but normal. I went to pieces.

I pictured them together. I burned with jealousy to think of them laughing and joking and having fun. It was May and the sun shone relentlessly, the hedgerows blossomed and the days lengthened into evenings warm enough to sit outside pubs by the river. The better the day, the worse I felt. In winter she would have been snuggled up under layers of thick sweaters but now she would be gliding about silkily in off-the-shoulder strappy tops and the shortest of shorts. Things I looked dreadful in. She was beautifully thin, lean-limbed and petite. And as time went on and the birds sang, I got worse. They were getting to know one another now, he was in love with her and they would be around town, arms entwined and he was giving me not even one passing thought. From the elation of having told him where to get off, after one lie too many and one letdown too intolerably far, I had sunk into the gloom of reality: he was gone and I would never see him again.

The depression immobilised me. I would stand in the middle of

Monica GRENFELL

a room and still be there twenty minutes later. I would stare at the ground, incapable of shifting my blank gaze onto anything more demanding than the pattern on the carpet. Even that was too much at times. Too busy, too much for my poor brain to cope with. For while my outer self was deep in despair and hopelessness, my inner world was in turmoil. What if this and why not that? How could I have had the car-crash of a relationship, how would I ever meet anybody again who even got near to him? My thoughts went round and round and always came back to the same place: I missed him and I wanted him back.

I stopped eating. I couldn't go to the gym. I could barely even go for a walk. From being a fit, strong and energetic woman I looked shrivelled and hollow. The demands on my body from a broken heart were literally taking it out of me. The pounding heart was impossible to bear and I would lie in bed listening to the loud thump-thump as I pondered the same thoughts over and over. How could I get over him? I lost 15lbs in three weeks.

Some women would kill to lose this much weight but of course it was 'weight' and not fat. My toned muscles went to pot. I lost vital fluids, due to not eating, and this is where most of the weight was lost. My nervous state was eating away at my lean tissue, giving me bad breath, spots and dull hair. Then after a month my heart changed one day. I wish I could say I got over my broken heart but far from it: I began to accept it.

When the reality of the situation hit home, the nerves were replaced by dullness. I began eating anything, at any time. Coupled with the inability to drag myself off the sofa, I began to spread. First my stomach and then my hips. I only gained maybe ten pounds but on my petite frame it could have been three stone: I looked like Michelin Man.

Then one day I woke up to myself. I would love to say I caught

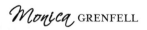

myself in the mirror and was disgusted, but I have never found shock tactics work and looking awful isn't an incentive as far as I am concerned. No, in fact it was a compliment I received. I went for a photo shoot and had a new make-up artist who hadn't known me before and so had nothing to compare me with. In my grief, I poured out the tale to explain why I looked so bad, and she stood back. Eyes wide open, head tilted to one side as she surveyed my face to make sure I wasn't displaying false modesty.

"But you're beautiful!" she exclaimed. "Beautiful and successful."
She put her hands to her hips and frowned.

"Are you having some sort of laugh?"

"No" I said. "I'm serious. I feel a frump, I have no confidence and he's out there enjoying himself with a girl twenty five years my junior – how can I compete?"

She shook her head and resumed her handiwork on my blotched complexion.

"Well all I can say is you're mad. You look fantastic to me. I had no idea of your age and I bet you he's out there thinking of you and wishing he was with you. He'd be mad not to. If you walked out of here and into him now, that's be the best revenge because he'd be kicking himself that he let you go"

Well, that was a stranger talking. It wasn't an obsequious friend or somebody I was paying. She didn't know me from Adam. And she thought he would regret ditching me if he met me now.

The Revenge diet was born

Monica GRENFELL

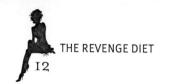

It is important that you put on a brave face and pretend that everything is all right with your world – even if it is not. It is easy to sink into depression and believe that nothing will ever go right for you again.

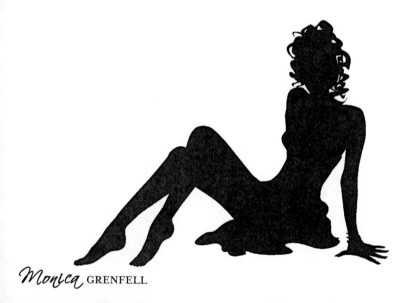

Monica GRENFELL

1. Wake Up! And change your PERSPECTIVE on
yourself

I bet all you want to do is cut to the chase and **skim right to the diet**. You don't want to be wasting time on psycho-babble and tedious ways to master motivation – all you want to know is what's for dinner tonight.

Then you're like the other 90% of the diet book-buying public – completely normal but completely doomed to shelling out for yet more diets and more unflattering clothes as you prop open the book and get writing your shopping list.

But hang on a moment –

Haven't you done that a dozen times before?

Didn't you skip the psycho-babble bits because you thought you knew it all?
Didn't you think the most important part of the book was what you got to EAT?

Well, that's where you went wrong. Tempting though it is to flip to the food, you need to read these next bits because THEY are the probably the reason you're overweight.

I know, you have personal triggers, like the fact he dumped you, the kids are causing mayhem and you have a sedentary job. Lots of

Monica GRENFELL

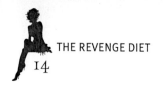
women tell me they only gained weight when they stopped playing tennis or took up computer work.

I believe them.

But hang on – I know people in wheelchairs who are thin! Being inactive in itself is no reason to get fat. And that's because, when it comes down to it, excess fat only collects in your body because you ate more than you needed.

And no other reason

Let's face it; most women are their own worst enemies when it comes to weight loss. We also tend to blame everything else on our failure to lose weight, insisting we're a 'special case' and that we were somehow meant to be fat.

Well, wake up !!

I have spent years – no, **decades** – listening to people who insist they cannot lose weight – and then seen them go on to do it. Not only that, but they never gained the weight back.

I am about to tell you the MAIN REASONS you're probably overweight and my key points for dealing with it once and for all. And at the same time addressing the points:

• Are diets and diet experts (like me!) just a waste of time and money and the only real solution is healthy eating?
• Is it better just to be curvy and happy?
• Should people accept you at face value and not judge you on your looks?

Monica GRENFELL

• And are men shallow and insensitive, unable to see beyond the outer, overweight shell to the beautiful person you are inside?

The reality is – nobody's 'right'. What matters is how you feel about the way you look and that you're willing to do what it takes to get your body back.

Yes, of course there are men who love bigger women. Of course there are lots of women who are fatter and happy. It goes without saying that people should accept you at face value and not judge you on your size.

But that's not the way of the world.

and

Truth No. 1!
Nothing will change about your body until you change your own behaviour.

Truth no. 2!
Blaming everything and everyone else for your weight problems won't shift a single ounce – it just puts off the day you do something and keeps you FAT for another day.

Truth no. 3!
Every minute you spend crying and depressed about your body or your lost love, your life is passing you by.

I'll deal with these truths in a minute, but for the moment you need

Monica GRENFELL

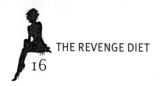
to move off the spot you're rooted to, stop feeling sorry for yourself, and take that first step:

Don't let him take everything!

It's easy to go to pieces. It can even be good to let it all out and allow yourself to grieve and feel sorry for yourself.

But remember:
- he's stolen your heart
- he's stolen your peace of mind
- Don't let him steal your looks as well!

Staying healthy doesn't just help you get through this: it shows the world that you care about yourself, haven't let yourself down and have plenty to offer.

Being slim and looking good will attract people to you and give you confidence, even if you are dying inside.

Say this to yourself when you don't feel like eating properly. Say this to yourself when you can't be bothered with the gym or having that healthy walk.

There is an upside – honestly!

You used to see him Tuesday and Saturdays. You spent every weekend with him. You lived with him! Whether you were full-on or part-time doesn't make any difference; suddenly you have yawning gaps in your life and frankly, if you're hurting and missing him, no time is good and you're probably pining twenty four hours a day.

But you have to stop thinking like that and start dealing with those times in a more positive way than just sitting there crying.

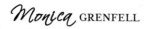

Monica GRENFELL

You don't have anywhere to go tonight?

Great!

You're staying in all weekend while your friends go out
and party?

Better still!!

You've got that week off work and should have been
going on holiday with him?

The Best!!!

By this time you're probably screaming that you don't need to hear
this. How can anything be good when you simply want to be with
him again?

OK you can go out with friends, but I'm not assuming you have an
entourage to turn to. You might just be Milly No-mates. I've been
that girl so I daresay you could be too.

Well, the good thing is you're not going anywhere and you have
what you've been craving all these years – TIME.

Suddenly you have hours to sit with face-masks, moisturising
cream on your legs and arms, conditioner on your hair.

You have time to plan and cook all those tempting, delicious little
meals you never had time for before.

In fact, you can turn your home into a health spa and spend the
entire week sipping iced rhubarb tea and nibbling celery salad if you
want. And if you have a love rival, just think:

She's the one stuffing herself with fattening food at romantic dinners right now – not you.

Monica GRENFELL

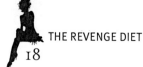

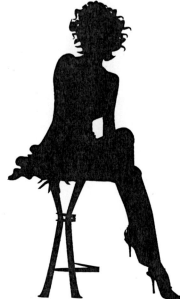

It is important that you make an effort to overcome your fears because if you don't you will be held back from doing something that could have been a lot of fun. The choice is simple: live up to your true potential or look back a few years from now and lament what might have been. You CAN make your dreams come true.

Monica GRENFELL

2. Things that get in the way: NEGATIVE thoughts

So let's assume you've got your head in a different place. Let's dwell on those negative thoughts for a moment and get them out of the way . . .

"Are diets and diet experts (like me!) just a waste of time and money and the only real solution is healthy eating?"

This is a great way to get yourself off the hook. You've found something else that doesn't work! Healthy eating is a wonderful idea but it won't make you slim by itself. Healthy food is like performance-enhancing drugs – they help people train better but they won't make them win races: otherwise your granny could take them and be an Olympic Gold medalist! The fact is, a healthy diet will help you to be healthy and low-calorie food will help you eat fewer calories, but the real key to being slim is . . .

Determination

If you are determined to be slim, you won't go near a biscuit until every last ounce has gone – and that's the truth of it.

Diet experts like me can only put a diet in place for you – but you need to be determined to follow it.

Nowadays we're faced by food everywhere we look, so restricting food takes effort. It is also not biologically natural to restrict our appetites. In fact, there is nothing to stop us eating ourselves to shapeless obesity except for one thing . . .

Monica GRENFELL

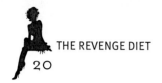
Vanity

That's right – vanity. We are the only animals who care what we look like and without vanity, who knows where we might be in terms of obesity? So when all the diets have been tried and the gym memberships have lapsed, self-control is all we've got.

Is it better just to be curvy and happy?

If 'curvy' is merely a euphemism for fat, forget it. If you are curvy and genuinely prefer yourself, fine. However, I have rarely met a woman who doesn't want to be thinner and there's a biological reason for this: we are creatures who display our assets in terms of fertility and availability. Larger breasts and hips certainly indicate fertility but a large waist and fat tum say "I might be pregnant – stay away!"

This is why a small waist is desirable to men. In any case, I have yet to meet a woman with a massive waist and big tummy who didn't wish they were smaller.

Should people accept you at face value and not judge you on your looks?

Sure, in an ideal world. I have many fat friends and family I love them all equally and don't care what their bodies look like as long as they're still my friends!

But seriously, this is an interesting point

People cannot evaluate what they cannot perceive. Just as you might think someone looks antagonistic or friendly or fierce or anxious, our bodies say something about us.

And however beautiful a person you are inside, nobody can see this and first impressions carry a lot of influence. Sorry, but this is the way of the world and nothing you can do will change it.

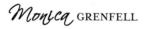

Monica GRENFELL

And are men shallow and insensitive, unable to see beyond the outer, overweight shell to the beautiful person you are inside?

No they're not. True, but most are not men are quite happy if their once-slim partner gains weight, but many are not. Whether you are offended by this is up to you, but ask yourself: would you be happy if the man you married stopped washing or shaving and turned into a smelly, fat and offensive slob? Would you accept it if he said you were being shallow just because you longer to see his toned physique again – the one you fell in love with?

Gaining weight and not doing something about it can be seen as an insult – saying "I really don't care what you think or how you like to see me." Who's insensitive now?

Stop the vicious circle

There are many ways in which you might be making your weight problems worse for yourself.

Happiness is contagious but it also doesn't attract attention.

And sadly, misery is often just another form of attention-seeking.

Other people, women in particular, might be nicer to you if you are fat

Just as they are nice to you if you are pregnant.

The reason?

You have ceased to be competition

Now, you might rail against this and insist that your friends love you for who you are and weight has nothing to do with it. If you don't believe me, lose weight and get a killer figure.

Monica GRENFELL

Notice how many of your friends start to say you look scrawny, gaunt or plain thin. In other words, they are afraid that you have started to be a threat.

So by staying fat, you are no threat and your friends can keep you in their circle.

Here are ways you might be making your weight worries worse:

- Looking for reassurance
- Monitoring and checking your weight constantly
- Finding out about slimming, reading magazines etc
- Avoiding things to do with being slim

Here's how to stop this vicious circle and start to diet successfully:

Stop asking for reassurance

We all need reassurance and love compliments. Talking over weight worries with friends and family can be very reassuring and make you relax for a time and eat that cake or takeaway without worry.

However too much reassurance means:

- You become preoccupied with your weight
- You stop believing the reassurance, needing more and more to reduce your worry as you see you are just as fat as before
- You look to others for reassurance, when it's more helpful to look to yourself.

More importantly, most people who are worried about their weight say reassurance doesn't work. Most of the time is makes things worse. And if you keep going to the doctor and clinics you might be sent for more unnecessary tests which make you more worried rather than less – especially when, inevitably, they come up with nothing.

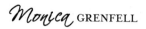

Monica GRENFELL

3. Welcome back –
to REAL dieting!

When I was a little girl, most women were on a diet. My mother, her sister, their friends: everyone.
'I'm slimming' they'd say. A week later, they'd lost those few pounds, so the deprivation didn't last long. Nowadays, people struggle with weight gain of three, four, five stone and more, and it can take months or even years to lose weight.

I guess women simply stayed on top of things better then. Clothes had to fit and you couldn't be going out buying new every time your waistband expanded. Bigger sizes weren't available. Nowadays you might ignore those few pounds, but in those days, without stretchy Lycra and other forgiving fabrics, an extra inch meant the zip wouldn't close and you had nothing to wear.

The whole sense of shape and figure was far more acute. Women cared because they had no choice. But in the process they looked good, kept their figures and nobody was fat!

With *The Revenge Diet*, I have brought back a sense of strict dieting without sacrificing nutrients. I think diets have become too liberal, as if the author is afraid of disappointing you as you trawl through the book trying to find out what you're going to eat.

- Most modern diets reassure you that you never need feel hungry

- Most modern diets provide food to 'fill you up'

- Most modern diets promise you never need feel hungry

Monica GRENFELL

But what they fail to do is tackle the reason you bought the book, which is to lose weight. In an effort to bury the negative, they fail to reinforce the positive — that you'll be thinner, fitter and more glamorous.

If you've been comfort-eating (and when did it ever bring you comfort?) the last thing you need is 'filling up'. In fact, you need **fewer** calories.

Comfort eating rarely brought anyone comfort for more than a few minutes, and more often it brings misery, discomfort and – fat.

SO in *The Revenge Diet*

1. I have cut calories to a realistically low level while boosting nutrition. You don't need calories if you want to shed bodyfat — the fat must work for you and act as your fuel.

2. I have increased the amount of dairy foods in the diet because as you'll read in a minute, dairy calcium has amazing properties to help you lose fat. Dairy foods are also more filling and nutritious than other carbohydrates and have the unique bonus of being 'complete foods'. This means milk and yogurt contain all three main nutrients, carbohydrate, fat and protein.

3. I have boosted nutrition. This means no 'fillers' of bread and cakes and 'healthy' snacks — you'll get all the healthy nutrients you need in far smaller portions than you probably thought.

For example, we all need about 55g protein a day. You get that in one small steak or half a pint of milk and a chicken breast.

We need 14mg iron which can be found in two bowls of cereal or a small portion of red meat. But you won't benefit from getting double the iron or protein by doubling portion size. You will just gain calories you don't need. So remember, when you eat for health

You can't be healthier than healthy!

This diet gives you what you need, in tasty meals and I promise:

- You will have more energy

- You will sleep better

- Your skin, hair and nails will grow healthily

- You won't feel bloated

- You will feel calmer

and don't forget

You're going to get thinner!

So let's get started on getting your body back and turning around this hopeless situation.

You WILL feel better soon – I promise!!

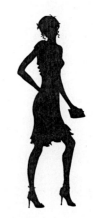

Monica GRENFELL

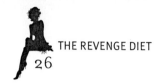
True Stories

Julie's story

I married quite late and had children when I was nearly 40. Having had the career thing, I was happy to embrace domesticity; I was dubious about giving up my job but my husband, Steve, said he'd support me all the way and it would be good to start a completely new life. We had three beautiful daughters, now aged 12, 9 and 7.

I certainly didn't let myself go – I'll say that from the start. I'd had a fabulous job in Public Relations and never had a hair out of place. Admittedly, I didn't wake up and climb into my killer heels once the children came along, but who does?

I guess I put a few pounds on – though it was more untoned muscles than acres of flab. I never had time for much exercise with three children, even though I always had good intentions. Children demand a lot of your time. None of this impacted on Steve anyway – he walked straight in and straight out to the gym every evening.

Writing that makes me cry. He wasn't at the gym; he was having an affair. To my shame, I'd always sneered at women who said they didn't suspect their husbands of having affairs or didn't notice the warning signs, but when my shock came, it was like an earthquake. Not only had Steve been having an affair, but he'd been having it since our youngest, Chloe, was born seven years ago. My whole world shattered.

I expected Steve to be contrite. I expected him to say it was nothing. I thought he'd ask forgiveness and beg me to let him stay. I pictured myself throwing him out and him saying he'd do anything to make amends to me and the girls and me eventually relenting and a happy ending.

Not a bit of it.

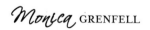
Monica GRENFELL

He said was that he'd fallen in love with one of his students and he was leaving me for her. He said I wasn't the woman he married. He said I wasn't the exciting sexy girl he fell for fourteen years ago. Then he made it worse by saying she was twenty years younger than me, willowy and blonde. He actually told me that. He told me she had the longest legs he'd ever seen and lips to die for. He said I'd got fat and had ignored his warning signs. What warning signs? He never said a word. If he'd ever for one second, suggested that I was getting fat I'd have done something about it. But he didn't. He reassured me time and again that I was still slim and lovely. In fact, he used to say he didn't know how I did it.

Can you believe this? Can you believe a man would be so cruel when you've done nothing but love him and care for him all these years, and bring up his children, that he could simply turn round and regale you with all these attributes of his stunning new girlfriend? A girl who'd done nothing for him but be good between the sheets.

I was in shock. He came for Sunday lunch. He took the girls swimming. If I'm being honest, I tried to stay calm so I didn't put him off. I mean, I knew he'd left me, and all my friends told me to kick him out and really make a scene. They told me to say he's not welcome, that I was finished with him and he could pack his bags and never come back. But I was clinging to some forlorn kind of hope that it wouldn't last between him and the girl and he'd remember that I was nice to him and no bridges were burned. I guess I simply wanted to be there for him, just in case. He was all I had; I loved him and felt lonely in bed.

But the weeks went by. He came round less often. I started selling the house so we could get divorced. Packing all my things after fourteen years simply tore me to bits. This had been my dream, the thing I'd given up a great job for. He'd taken me from a comfortable world, married me, given me three children and left. I know I should

Monica GRENFELL

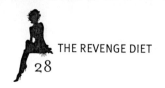
be positive and thank him for the girls and take my share of the blame. But I wasn't. I became bitter and twisted.

I remember lying in bed talking to the ceiling. For hours I regaled the empty space with questions and accusations and bitterness. I asked him why he hadn't told me, why he hadn't said he was unhappy. I asked him how he could do this to me. I asked what on earth I and our wonderful little girls had ever done to him except love him and care for him. I asked if she greeted him back from work with a cosy kitchen and three bright-eyed, smiling little girls' faces. I asked endless questions, always ending up with me dissolving into tears once again.

I would go shopping and be OK. I would have days of immense calm. Then out of the blue, great jags of crying would rip through me. How could he do this? How can one person have such an effect on another?

I piled on the weight. I stopped caring what I looked like,. I gained ten and then twenty pounds. Soon it was forty. My face was bloated and my thighs like tree-trunks. I was such a total mess; I wouldn't be there when he came round. I hid myself away and cried. And cried and cried.

Then one day I met a friend who hadn't known of the split. She was a fun girl. I told her the long story. "What if you run into the girl?" she laughed. "I bet he's told her all sorts about you. I bet he's painted you as fat and plain and said you never had sex together. She's only young, don't forget. However self-assured she might appear, she's a lot younger than you. Shock her. And while she's shocked she'll have a bash at him and you're home and dry. Or at least if you're not home and dry, he won't be living in his cosy little world any more. "

She got me thinking. I hadn't pictured this.

I was asked to test *The Revenge Diet*. I only did it with great reluctance because Monica said I was miserable anyway, so I might as well be miserable trying to get somewhere as miserable doing nothing. I can't say it made any sense to me at the time, but now it's obvious. You have to keep on living, so you might as well stay alive trying to get a better life than being sunk in a bad life. The days pass just the same.

Losing the first ten pounds cheered me more than winning the lottery. I mean that. Looking slimmer is a huge incentive. By the time I'd lost fifteen pounds in four weeks, I felt as if my entire life had been transformed. It wasn't just the fact of being slimmer; I'd been eating any old rubbish and suddenly I was consuming foods that helped my brain functions and my moods to improve. I stopped eating erratically and stuck to three meals a day. My starchy dinner helped me to sleep so I could wave goodbye to the dreaded eye bags. I would love to say I turned the clock back and I suddenly looked ten years younger but something better happened: I stopped caring whether I did or didn't.

I felt great. I felt confident. I went to the gym and joined a jive class. Soon I was proficient and had met two fantastic blokes who danced so sexily I looked back on my husband and couldn't believe I had spent so long with him. I couldn't believe I'd been pining for him. Less than a year had passed since he walked out and I didn't care. I certainly didn't want him back.

I now have a great boyfriend and as soon as the divorce is through, we're getting married. I'd love to say my husband's relationship ended or is going through a bad patch but to tell the truth, I don't know and I don't care. He's out of my life and out of my mind. I love my new man, he loves the girls and all I know is my breakup was the golden opportunity for a second bite of the cherry. I'm still on *The Revenge Diet* because it suits me and I know I'm taking care of my looks. But sad to say, I'll never be able to take a man for granted any more – I'll always be glancing over my shoulder.

Monica GRENFELL

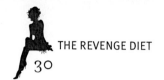
4. The Secret SUCCESS of the Revenge Diet

The two main secrets of success in this diet are:

1. When you eat – and
2. The role of dairy calcium in fat loss.

But let's not get ahead of ourselves . . .

It is important to eat to your bodyclock. For years, people have been doing high-protein, very low carbohydrate diets to lose weight and cutting carbohydrates in the evening in the misguided belief that calories eaten in the evening somehow make you fatter than at any other time of day.

This is from the idea that the food you eat has to be 'burned off' . . .

Not true!

Food provides calories and calories fuel your body all the time. In fact our greatest calorie expenditure is in doing absolutely nothing. We burn calories day and night, only sometimes we burn them more quickly and sometimes more slowly. Like a massive power plant, our bodies are never switched off. Sometimes your body runs slowly, like when you're asleep, and sometimes it runs at full capacity, such as when you're stressed, working hard and dashing about. Food's purpose is to provide calories but it also feeds and nourishes, maintains and repairs your body.

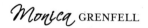

You see, carbohydrate stores go straight to your muscles (and liver) as energy stores and this is like watering a parched plant or holding a dry sponge under a tap and watching it absorb the water. Your muscle stores hold water and this is why, when people go back to 'normal' eating after a diet they might find they gain weight fast.

High protein diets drain the stored energy from your muscles so you actually lose weight quite quickly.

But most of it is water, not fat.

And the REAL problem is that after a short time you simply can't stay away from those lovely baked potatoes, curries and pasta dishes!

Well, I don't think you need to.

The food to avoid in the evening is PROTEIN. Meat, cheese and chicken take several hours to be digested, so eating them in the evening can result in bloating and discomfort as you struggle to sleep while food is churning inside.

Starchy carbohydrates, on the other hand, are digested far more quickly. Plus, you need to store energy for the following day so you wake up refreshed and lively, not woolly and confused!

The beauty of dairy

Dairy foods are the cornerstone of great looks and health. If you don't tolerate dairy (and this is rare) you may have soya milk and yogurt and soya cheese. However, as you are about to discover, dairy calcium has particular benefits in weight-loss diets, especially fat loss in the abdomen.

The link between dairy calcium and fat loss was first established over

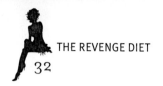
twenty years ago. However a recent study found some exciting new evidence which I hope will turn you on to dairy food all the more.

The study

Dr Michael Zemel and co-workers' study *'Calcium and Dairy Acceleration of Weight and Fat Loss during Energy Restriction in Obese Adults'* Results indicate that those who included 3 portions of dairy products (milk, yogurt and cheese) as part of a calorie-controlled diet lost more weight and fat than those who consumed 1 portion of dairy a day or less. The fat loss was particularly significant in the trunk area.

This human intervention study is the first clinical trial to directly compare the weight loss effects of reduced-calorie diets high in calcium from dairy to those high in calcium from supplements.

The 32 obese adults followed one of three diets (all of which were 500 calories lower than their normal calorie intake) for 24 weeks:

- Diet high in dairy – at least 3-4 portions of milk, cheese or yogurt each day.
- Diet high in calcium from supplements, but low in dairy.
- Diet low in calcium and low in dairy.

Results

The adults on a reduced-calorie diet who ate 3 portions of dairy products each day lost significantly more weight and body fat (particularly from the trunk area) than those on the other diets.

		GROUP DIET AVERAGE % WEIGHT LOSS	AVERAGE % FAT LOSS	AVERAGE % FAT LOSS IN TRUNK AREA
HIGH DAIRY	Total calcium intake 1200–1300mg of calcium each day.Consumed 3 – 4 portions of milk, cheese or yogurt.	10.9%	14.1%	14.0%
HIGH CALCIUM FROM SUPPLEMENTS, LOW DAIRY	Total calcium intake of 1200 –1300mg of calcium each day. Consumed no more than 1 portion of dairy a day and an 800mg calcium supplement.	8.6%	11.6%	12.9%
LOW CALCIUM, LOW DAIRY	Total calcium intake of 400 – 500mg of calcium each day. Consumed no more than 1 portion of dairy a day and a placebo supplement.	6.4%	8.1%	5.3%

How significant is this study?

A growing body of scientific evidence suggests that including low-fat dairy products as part of a calorie-controlled diet may help with weight loss.

The study suggests that dieters should think twice before limiting their dairy intake. Eating three portions of dairy each day may help to keep weight down by encouraging fat to be burnt rather than stored.

Monica GRENFELL

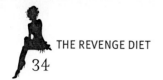
When to eat

Should you eat nothing after 6pm? Or 5pm? How about carb curfews?

Well, I'll tell you something about these ideas:

These are all TOTAL MYTHS that I really, really want to dispel in this book.

This is when and what to eat:

1. After a night's sleep

Have a major meal (in terms of quality, not a massive amount) You are empty, you haven't eaten for maybe ten hours and you need to top up. Have protein at this meal, with non-starchy carbs like fruit or milk. Protein will keep you full for longer than carbohydrates.

My recommendations are eggs and orange juice, the perfect combination of protein and carbohydrates.

2. Middle of the day

You need a very light, protein-based but carbohydrate-light meal like cheese and fruit with nuts. Never eat much at lunchtime if you're on a diet and never have snacks. You might feel hungry but this mustn't swerve your resolve: if you have excess fat, you must go between meals without a snack. Remember, it isn't a full stomach you need, but a nourished body. As long as you get your day's requirements of nutrients , you must not keep adding calories for the sake of it.

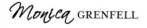

3. In the evening

You should eat a high carbohydrate, low protein meal at this time of day. I call this 'stocking the supermarket shelves after the store has closed'. They don't stock up as customers come in to start buying. And this is how you should think of your energy stores: filled up the night before so you can sleep well, your blood sugar levels are nice and high and your body can relax, rest and repair itself while you sleep.

I know you'll be thrilled with this diet, which will help you lose loads of weight and get your body and looks back.

But unfortunately, before we really get going, you're going to have to trawl through more bad stuff – the bits where you face your failings and beat yourself up over all the things you've done wrong in your diet! It's sad, but it's necessary because 80% of the problem isn't what you've been eating but the excuses you've made for not getting to grips with yourself before now. But hopefully, at the end of this programme you'll turn a new leaf, get that situation out of your system and – make him truly sorry he lost you!!

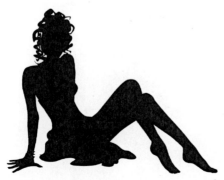

Monica GRENFELL

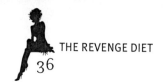

Don't waste time or energy on people who seem to believe that you exist merely to fulfill their needs and wishes. If they really do think like that then they deserve neither your support nor your affection. Others may take you for granted but you must never buy into the lie that you are second rate. You're simply the best.

Monica GRENFELL

5. The dieter's worst enemy – HERSELF

Have you ever looked at a tub of ice cream or a whole packet of biscuits and after pausing a second, slammed straight into them, eating every last bit?

Have you done this, despite knowing you were over-weight and supposed to be dieting?

In your mind, you knew what you were doing would keep you fat, make you feel bad and put you back even further than you were before, due to overpowering GUILT at being so greedy.

Another one...

Have you ever woken up with every intention of going to the gym, then had one more coffee, settled down under the duvet for just ten more minutes – and then given up because it was all too late now? Honestly, have you ever had this happen?

Of course, the worst part wasn't that it happened, but that you KNEW it would happen . . . and you did it anyway.

And finally . . .

Have you ever been clothes shopping with your man, tried on several items knowing you were too big for

Monica GRENFELL

them or looked dreadful . . . and moaned and complained and gone home in tears . . . maybe your boyfriend said something about your weight once but your eyes glazed over and you complained to your girlfriends he had the NERVE to mention it? And maybe he became distant from you — and the relationship ended soon after?

You were trying to CONVINCE yourself that you looked ok and possibly even compare yourself favourably with someone who was even bigger than you . . .

I'm guessing that when one of these things happened, your girlfriends said things like:
"That weight suits you"

Or they said:
"He's an idiot – how dare he mention your weight!"

Or even
"You're curvy – who wants to be like these stick-thin, anorexic models anyway?"

And then one day you see that they're thin themselves and maybe they've even run off with your man – well, it happens.

And the worst part of all: You kept eating the ice cream.

The main PROBLEM here, and the thing that stood in your way, is that just because your girlfriends told you it wasn't your fault, doesn't mean that they **understood** the problem.

The people who try to comfort and encourage you have good intentions. They're just trying to make you feel better.

But without realising it, they're making the situation WORSE.

They're trying to blame the situation on HIM, (for not loving you fat) on society, (for being 'fattist') on clothes manufacturers (for not getting sizing right or skimping on material or designing clothes for skinny people – add your own excuse here . . .) instead of trying to help you understand how to get and keep a good figure.

Food – love or hate?

You might convince yourself you love food – and love of food is standing in your way of success and slimness.

But people who say they love food, often hate it. You're fixated and obsessed – and making things worse for yourself.

See if I'm right by asking yourself:
- Does your weight dominate your life?
- Do you bury yourself in slimming magazines?
- Do you return to slimming clubs again year after year?
- Do your conversations with friends mostly centre on weight?
- Do you have mostly fat friends?
- Do you automatically scorn slim celebrities?
- Do you say healthy food is boring?
- Do you automatically check calories and fat grams on labels?
- Do you blame your weight on emotional or medical problems?
- Do you insist that diets don't work?

If you answered 'yes' to more than five questions, you aren't in control any more and you have no power over your mind – in fact, food does.

Monica GRENFELL

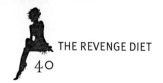

So start with small steps:

• Give up the slimming clubs

This links you emotionally with your problem. Slimming groups are good and give support to people who need to lose weight and deal with their problems once or twice. If you're a yo-yo dieter, however, this type of club is useless – centred on meals, calories, fat and other nutritional matters, they are wrong for you.

Your RELATIONSHIP with food is the issue – it's the reason you're in pain.

• Give up the habit of choosing and checking your food and buying special slimming ranges.

Food is your enemy! Not all food, but we're talking about overeating.

To get power back, kick the entire problem out of your life.

Remove all traces of your addiction – special recipes, low-calorie foods.

• Stop the therapy.

You can spend hours talking about how your break-up or PMT made you overeat.

You can spend months trying to understand why you overeat.

But you know what happens?
• After a while your friends will walk away.
• They'll talk about you as boring and avoid you.
• They'll even say your misery is attention-seeking.

You're fat because you ate too much. You must face this.

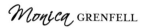

• Stop the cycle

We all need reassurance and compliments. Talking over weight worries with friends and family can be very helpful and make you relax for a time and eat that cake or takeaway without worry.

However too much reassurance means:
• You become preoccupied with your weight
• You stop believing the reassurance, needing more and more to reduce your worry as you realise you're just as fat as before
• You look to others for reassurance, when it's more helpful to look to yourself.

More importantly, most people who are worried about their weight say REASSURANCE DOESN'T WORK. Most of the time it makes things worse. And if you keep going to the doctor and clinics you might be sent for more unnecessary tests which make you more worried rather than less – especially when, inevitably, they come up with nothing.

Instead

• It's OK that you need support, but get it by doing different things and associating with fit people.

• Remove the power of food by giving your attention to something else

• Decide not to talk about weight or food for a month. If friends ask you, don't get sucked in. Change the subject.

• Remove yourself to a place where food isn't an issue, like the library.

Monica GRENFELL

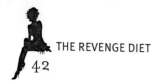
- For a month, refuse all invitations where there's temptation

- Eat boring stuff. If you were really hungry, you'd snack on hard-boiled eggs or cold meat, right? Eat three plain meals a day and nothing in between. Never eat unless you're at a table. Buy food fresh each day. Have weird combinations like scrambled eggs and peas that aren't exciting but are actually good food that nourishes you. Lose your relationship with your enemy by not loving it!

- Don't carry money around when you go for a walk. If you can't buy it, you can't eat it.

- Don't go round with unhealthy people who scoff at good habits.

- Never associate with people who think bingeing, smoking or drinking are fun topics.

AND REMEMBER:

You aren't a victim, you're a winner.

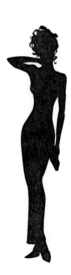

Monica GRENFELL

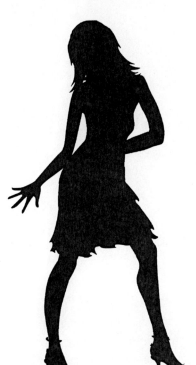

Going on a diet might be the best thing that ever happened to you. Instead of thinking 'it's tough' think of the freedom you'll get from torment. Food has too much place in your mind – fill that space with thoughts of slimness and take whatever you have to do as a positive step.

Monica GRENFELL

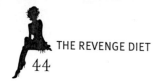

6. The SIX DEADLY MISTAKES people make without ever realising it . . .

Through my research and personal experience, I've found that these six mistakes are responsible for more weight problems, failed diets and broken relationships than any other factors.

Here they are:

Mistake no. 1 – Deciding on failure

Some women think of their figures as complete injustices. Spending their lives punishing themselves with diets, they treat themselves as walking laboratories for every new fad and flavour-of-the-month diet that comes along. But the real problem is deciding they can't be successful or that somehow they were born to be fat.

This is where you fall down. Don't get caught up in the negative, and what's wrong with your weight: whatever it is, it can be changed.

Most people focus on the downside of taking control of their lives.

They say 'what if this happens and what if that happens?' People get caught up in worry about being hungry. So instead of accepting this, they take every possible precaution that they have enough food to hand instead of thinking that food has been their problem all along. Then they move towards those negative thoughts and nothing happens and they stay fed up and static.

Monica GRENFELL

But if you make a positive thing your goal, like losing weight or getting firmer thighs, you will move towards that, and each day you're that tiny bit further.

And it's like when your hair grows – you can't see each millimetre and maybe a month goes by – but each day it's growing a bit more.

Then how about the fact that a diet is unpleasant? It's not unpleasant but you start to focus on that. How many other, everyday things are not so pleasant but we do them? The rain? Getting up night after night to a crying baby? What about standing in line at the supermarket or waiting for a bus? They aren't pleasant. But we don't complain every time these things happen.

Mistake no. 2 – Insisting that 'Nothing works'

It's like this: you have a car – a very fast, top-of-the-range car, like a Ferrari. Is it fast? Of course it is. But what if your old granny drives it? Or it sits on your driveway with a full tank of petrol and nobody behind the wheel? Is it fast then?

A cake recipe doesn't guarantee you'll get a perfect cake. You can line up ten people with the same ingredients and the same recipe, but each cake will be different. Why did her cake rise while yours is a flop? Nobody knows. But do you say "I'm never making that cake again", or do you try again and maybe tweak a bit one way and adjust another and suddenly after three tries you have a perfect cake!

And I bet you wouldn't say the recipe was useless just because your first cake didn't turn out right. Right?

Monica GRENFELL

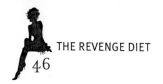
Mistake no. 3 – Looking for the get-out clause

Some diet clubs give you a list of 'treats'. They also give you a food allocation and allow for extra food if you exercise and systems for saving food for another day. You are constantly bargaining and rewarding yourself with the very thing that got you into the mess in the first place. Rewarding yourself with chocolate is not a treat for your body. A treat for your body would be an apple, a few grapes or a piece of fish.

Respect your body by never again allowing any rubbish inside it. Never eat meals that come from some factory. You get out what you put in, and the rewards will be a fat-free, lean, energetic and healthy shape.

Mistake no. 4 – Lack of discipline

In case you were just groaning and mentally listing all the reasons you can't possibly be disciplined, I bet you're already a pretty disciplined person anyway.

- You get up and go to work
- You take exceptional care of your hair
- You never go without a manicure
- You'd rather die than have a messy kitchen
- Your clothes are always immaculate
- You keep up with friends religiously.
- If you say you'll be somewhere at ten, you will be.

You can probably think of a few more!

The point is, we're all lazy about something. I'm lazy about the ironing. Every week, I promise myself that I'll stay on top next time and iron things as they come along.

Monica GRENFELL

But I never do. That old pile simply gets bigger and my stress piles up along with it. But I know one thing: if I suddenly had a call and friends were turning up out of the blue, I'd clear that ironing in a flash!

And that brings me to one major truth about slim women or weight loss.

You need a compelling reason.

Ever noticed that women can usually lose weight for their wedding? Or a holiday?

If you're drifting from day to day, even if your life is good and full, without a compelling reason to be slim, you probably won't get on and do it. You'll tell yourself each day that you'll start that diet, then by the time the biscuits emerge at elevenses, you'll give in saying 'one won't hurt' and then it's two or three and you'll think "there's always tomorrow".

Pull yourself together!

All this time you're bargaining with your idle nature, time is ticking. You'll never have this day again. And I'll tell you something else: I have met hundreds of women in their forties and fifties and older, who regret bitterly the time they wasted when they were young, not getting to grips with their weight, so they spent their youth fat. And now they're older and it seems too late.

Well, it's NEVER too late.

Monica GRENFELL

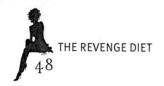
Are you going to let another year go by while you cry bitter tears about your weight? Remember why you wanted this.

Mistake no. 5 – Living in denial

Nobody ever just woke up fat. Nobody eats a slice of chocolate cake, looks down and their hips are three inches wider. Despite what everyone says about certain foods being 'fattening' there's no evidence of this. Hey, you just had a wild night out, drunk yourself into the ground and had a takeaway and guess what – you're still the same weight and your clothes still fit!!

Well of course they do. You can't see your hair growing either. But you know it's longer than two days ago.

If you are overweight, it came from somewhere. Somewhere along the line you must have gained two, then five then ten pounds.

And that's how weight 'creeps on'. After a while, you don't go on the scales. Insisting you're 'happy with your weight' you decide to lose a few pounds before you learn the truth. But days go by, you can always start tomorrow and you start convincing yourself you can't expect to be slim after a baby/ the age of forty/your recent illness (fill in your own excuse once again).

This is total denial and you know what? – it's stressful and makes matters worse.

And you know this is true!

Mistake no.6 – Concentrating on FOOD and EATING

What's the first thing someone does when they embark on a new diet? Sort out their food.

Monica GRENFELL

They write lists, head for the supermarket with the largest trolley imaginable and fill it to the brim with – food. OK it's healthy stuff, like fruit, vegetables, fish and chicken. They're going to need it and after all, you can give up cigarettes and alcohol but you can't give up food, they say.

Fair enough.

But this is the first thing they've done wrong and I bet you do it too.

Concentrate on eating

Food is your downfall. You either eat carelessly, thoughtlessly, indiscriminately, you gorge, binge, pick, indulge . . . whatever approach you take, it's still all down to eating. And this has been your problem all along.

A client with a severely broken heart, who is crying all the time and barely hanging on . . . said to me the other day

"I just about manage to swerve the chocolate these days . . . if this was a year ago I would have gone straight to it in my distress, but now I reach for the carrot sticks instead"

Is this OK?   NO!

I'll tell you why.

My client has a hand-to-mouth response to stress. We all have it: it's natural and it means the body is trying to fuel itself up in anticipation of a physical crisis.

You feel stress: your body releases fat cells so you have enough fuel for the fight . . . and the response is to put more food into your body to make up for it.

Monica GRENFELL

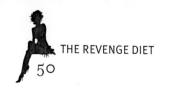
Some people chew pencils or their nails. Some people smoke. Others chew gum.

But most people reach for food.

Remember, you're not about to run for your life or tackle a lion. The stress response has no outlet and those fat cells go back, not to where they came from, but to your abdomen. But that's another story.

The problem with replacing sugary snacks with carrot sticks is that it does nothing to train you out of the habit. You feel stress: you eat.

But one day you won't have the carrots. All there'll be are sweets or crisps or a local convenience store, inconveniently selling biscuits. Unable to resist your habit, you lay into them.

Bad habit!

Here's another one:

You go out, see an outfit you love, struggle with your conscience for a second, then take it to the till. You have to have it!

You're wavering, but you flash the credit card. Transaction done.

But imagine if you had to go home and bring back the cash, and home is twenty minutes away? How likely is it that you'll buy the dress?

80% of people wouldn't buy it. The distance between wanting and having is too great. It involves effort and inconvenience. But credit cards bring the distance between desire and fulfillment to a few minutes; not really enough time to change your mind.

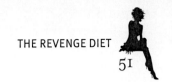

Ok, you can take it back. But how likely is that?

The moral of this story applies to food. Here, then are my three GOLDEN RULES for dealing with these tricky times:

Golden rule 1
Never eat as a response to stress.

Think this is easier said than done? Imagine if you had a peanut allergy. You'd have no trouble avoiding them!

So it IS possible to stay your hand and think again. You know it's possible and there's no such thing as 'can't help myself'. You can!

Golden rule 2
Put a distance between you and the object of your downfall.

Always buy food daily where possible, and certainly NEVER have fattening, junky food 'in' just in case someone drops by. They never do and if they did, would you really give them sweets and crisps?
  By keeping your cupboards bare, you're helping them as much as helping yourself.

Change your attitude before you change your diet. Going into a new regime with your old thoughts means fighting against new food and your desires to eat the old stuff that made you fat. With a NEW attitude, you will think healthily and dare I say it –

Like a slim person.

Monica GRENFELL

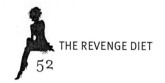
True Stories

Tanya's story

I'd been going out with John for ten months. He used to email every day and I emailed back. We lived a distance apart and only saw one another twice a week, but it was lovely. We knew instantly that we were soulmates and had a good time together. The one thing I remember was how well we got on and never had a bad moment.

He had a reputation as a womaniser. But that seemed all from the past as he was already 46. I was 29. I did ask him about rumours of his Bad Boy image but he said he was younger then and after all, what single man shouldn't go out with a lot of women? He also said that he'd lived with one girl for 5 years and another for three years, so that took care of some of his adult life. And he had never cheated while in a relationship.

To be fair, we broke up a couple of times over silly things. The breakups lasted a day in one case and a week the second time. It wasn't serious. But one day we broke up and he didn't instantly try and get back with me; he left me to do the running.

I contacted him after four weeks and simply told him I missed him. It was true: I'd been in utter misery. I realized that although things weren't perfect these glitches were nothing. We'd been madly in love and both thought we'd met our perfect partner. I was right to flounce off when I did, and even thought I'd be happier without him but soon realised I was better with him. I pined dreadfully.

We got back together. But something was wrong. He seemed too attentive, too eager to say there was nobody else in his life and I was the only woman he had round his house. I smelled a rat. Then he admitted it: He'd met someone else while we were on our 'break'

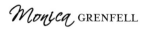

Monica GRENFELL

and while he ran her down dreadfully and said he didn't love her, he seemed only too keen to let her in when she came knocking.

He kept saying I was number one. But she kept drifting back and landing on his doorstep. I know I should have got out there and then but honestly the way he told it, she was practically stalking him. I would ask why, if she was such a nuisance he didn't simply tell her to sling her hook, and he'd say she was a nutter or she'd been crying or he simply gave her a bed in the spare room out of pity. I took the view that I would be there for him as I was his best bet, I adopted the air of a good listener and we continued to have great times and even greater sex.

The day the bombshell came was the worst of my life. He confessed to me that the girl was pregnant. He said he still didn't care about her, but he'd do the decent thing and stand by her. She lived a long way away and I know he didn't see her for six weeks at one stage. I reckoned I could just about put up with this as he was charm itself to me and vowed that I was the only one who understood him.

The end, when it came, was ugly. We'd just had a brilliant weekend but on the Monday I got a text saying "D. is back. See you soon I hope x" I texted back asking if she was there for good.

"Who knows" was the reply.

Then he asked if he could see me sometime.

He actually wanted to keep me going as his 'affair'! I was so brutally wounded, I can barely write this without sobbing. I sat at home crying, I was so bad I even gave up my job. I ate and ate, stupid things as if to punish myself. I got fat and my face got bloated. I lay in bed aching to have him hold me. The physical longing to have sex with him was a pain I'll never forget. Funnily enough I slept, because I'd stay awake until 2am just watching TV or drinking, so I guess it was more a case of passing out than sleeping. But as soon as I woke, I'd cry. My stomach heaved with grief. Despite him being the worst kind of rat, I missed everything about him. I still do.

Monica GRENFELL

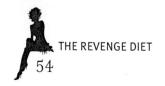

Picturing them in bed together was torture. And it's no good saying go out and have fun and meet new people – I didn't want new people. I didn't enjoy so-called fun because I missed him being with me. No man matched up. Can you believe that – that after all that time and all the letdowns, this rat had exceeded all expectations and been the Bad Boy he always said he was? At least he didn't lie about that.

I did crazy things. Near my home was a hill and from that hill you could see a long distance, ten miles at least. And there was a landmark, a cluster of trees on the hillside above his town, and you could see it from the top of the hill. Every evening, I would walk up the hill, a walk of maybe half an hour. It was high and windy and desolate. And I would stare across ten miles to that landmark and know that somewhere there, somewhere in the town below was his house. In his house he'd be sitting with her, perhaps she'd have her legs flung across his as I used to do. Perhaps the fire would be burning or she'd be cooking dinner. Even if he was out at the pub it was there, below those trees, in that town. Every night I climbed that hill like some deranged idiot, demented with grief, and I stood looking at some distant place on the landscape where he lived and sobbed my heart out.,

I don't know what made me go on a diet. I was at rock bottom. I couldn't go any further. It gave me something to do I suppose. I thought I was bad enough so I couldn't get any worse. I was smoking a lot and that had to stop. In an act of almost inhuman masochism, I decided to give up cigarettes and food at the same time. Not all food of course, but the junk I was eating my way through, torturing myself with failure and making myself hideous.

The Revenge Diet was the only thing that worked for me because it was strict. I wasn't in any sort of shape to be making decisions from long lists of meals. I couldn't be doing with calculations and

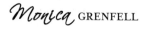

adding up calories or something. I just wanted to prop up the diet and go.

I lost all the weight I gained and a little bit more. I'm now 8 stone and 5ft 2ins which is right for my petite frame. The best bit is my hair looks fabulous and my skin is getting great comments. It's very sheeny which I guess is from the fish and nuts. Anyway, I saw him the other day. He was pushing a pram and the flashy car had given way to a family saloon with a child seat in the back. He saw me too and we had a few words. He didn't look happy and I could tell he felt trapped. By sheer good chance I'd just been for a manicure and had coloured my hair the day before and I knew I looked good. To be honest, I'd been walking around every single day with my good clothes and hair done in case I saw him and I never did. But this time it paid off and it sort of cured me. Yes, he looked good. Yes, I could probably get him back. I even have a feeling he'll call me . . . But he looked at me that day with utter shell-shock and I could tell he fancied me. Since then, that grinding ache in my stomach has vanished. I don't feel permanently panicked. He fancied me and maybe he wanted to take me to bed and I know that he never will.

And that, to be honest, is all I really wanted".

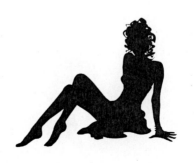

Monica GRENFELL

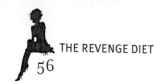
Make a point of focusing on the positive things in your life, the things that bring you joy. It's your mind that creates your reality, so make sure your thoughts are cheerful

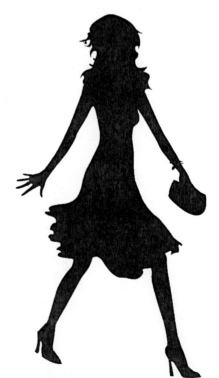

Monica GRENFELL

7. The Secret to LOSING WEIGHT and keeping it off forever

Setting goals –

So we're about to embark on the diet. You set goals and this makes you feel great. But then you sit back and wait for something to happen. And you know what?

Nothing happens.

Setting goals is fine. But you need to achieve them and that means having a STRATEGY.

Goals have to be measurable. It's no good saying you want to go from here to there — and then leave it at that. You must plot it like you plan a journey. It's like saying you want to go from Southampton to Scotland and then just drive there without planning your route. The route in this case is this diet, but in the past you might have gone another route, like calorie-counting or lowfat or high-fibre; fine if they got you there and you enjoyed the journey. But sometimes you need to try a different route.

You also need to measure your progress. Along the way you'll be making stops and on those stops you might get out the map again

Monica GRENFELL

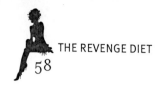
and see how far you've gone and check traffic warnings and maybe change direction or plan to arrive earlier or later. (I'm beginning to love this journey analogy!)

The stops in this case are your weigh-ins. And during these times that you can change course, decide on other courses of action to steer you out of trouble or simply see that you're doing OK and can carry on the journey as planned.

So you say:
- Am I losing weight?
- If not, why not?
- Could I be a little more disciplined?
- Could I cut portion sizes down a little?
- Am I burning enough calories through exercise?

This might all seem a lot right now, but as you progress, I guarantee it'll become a way of life. And as you lose weight, shape up and start to see that lovely figure once again, you'll see the point of it all.

Make this simple pledge to yourself: this is the last day you will feel and look like this.

Your luck will turn . . . and you must be ready when it does.

Ask yourself how many times in the past you have let opportunities pass you by. Now ask yourself if you are going to do the same thing again.

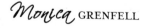

Many of the things you have been worrying about are simply not worth the effort. Focus only on positive ideas and positive news – and your positive attitude will renew your world.

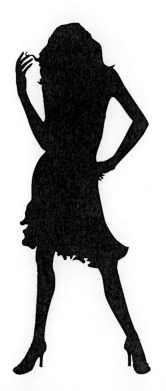

Monica GRENFELL

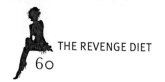
8. Getting your BODY back!

Let's not forget why you're doing this. That guy dumped you. Your husband walked out. Something happened and you're hurting: you probably let yourself go through drinking and smoking too much.

So you have
- A stressed liver through too much alcohol
- Stressed insulin through too much sugar and processed food
- Stressed skin through lack of vitamins and water
- Too much fat packed round vital organs and between muscle fibres
- Poor bone density

These things can ALL be remedied with the right diet and exercise, and it doesn't take long. In fact, you'd be amazed how quickly you can turn yourself around and on this programme.

Yes, sitting for hours with girlfriends, sharing a Chinese takeaway a bottle of wine and two packets of cigarettes helped at the time

But where did they get you, really?

Be kind to yourself. Getting fat and bloated is heaping pain on pain, failure on failure. You might not get him back or even want him back. You might not have done any of the things I just mentioned. You've probably kept yourself together remarkably intact, yet your heart is still breaking. And you know something – this is as damaging to your looks as overeating and drinking. Stress and heartbreak take a terrible toll on the body.

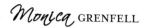
Monica GRENFELL

You might not be able to control your tears right now, and might just be holding up. I understand that, and I'm not going to tell you to simply 'move on'. If you could do that, you'd have done it. But I can help you manage the physical stress.

And this will make you feel so much better.

Your body is the only one you have; you cannot take a weekend break from it, divorce it, fall out with it or take a sabbatical. You live inside your body so it makes sense to try and get along.

And this body of yours might have to last eighty years which is a long time to maintain it and keep in good condition.

Think of your body like some amazing processing plant, a huge engine room which is dedicated to the long-term job of not just keeping you alive, but managing all the things you do from day-to-day.

For example:
- making blood
- transporting waste
- Processing food
- Extracting nutrients to feed skin, hair and nails and all other growth processes.
- Repairing worn and used muscles
- Making new muscle fibres,
- Strengthening and reinforcing bone
- Regulating your temperature.
- Regulating your hormones round the clock

Need I go on?

Monica GRENFELL

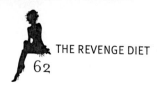

In the time it has taken to read this page, several million cells have died and new ones have been made. And like any engine, you need fuel for these processes.

I'm confident you'll achieve
- 15lbs Weight loss in four weeks
- Improved sleep
- Relief from constipation
- A Flatter tummy
- Smoother skin and less cellulite

Metabolism

what is it, can it be ruined by years of weight gain and loss and if I can't lose weight, is it just because I have a slow metabolism?

Metabolism is described as the energy cost of maintaining the body. In other words, respiration, nerve and muscle tone and circulation.

So you're like a car in some ways – sometimes you're running as if you just turned the key and your engine is idling and sometimes you're going at full pelt on the motorway with all systems stretched.

Metabolism is also based on how heavy your body is and how much is lean tissue. So to go back to the car analogy, a mini goes a long way on a tank of petrol because it's small and a Rolls Royce only does a few miles on a tank because it's huge.

So – sorry to say . . .

The larger you are, the higher your metabolic rate.

Monica GRENFELL

But

It depends on what is making you larger. Is it muscle, fat or a mix of both?

Muscle is what's called metabolically active. This means muscles are active all the time.

Fat simply sits there, doing nothing.

Forget those lame tips about chilies or drinking green tea or a hot curry raising your metabolism – they don't.

Muscle governs your metabolic rate.

So the more you have, the more calories your body will need each day and – *yessss!* – The more food you can eat without gaining weight.

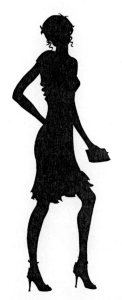

Monica GRENFELL

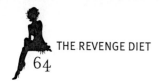
Your hardworking body

Every minute of the day, your body is working hard. Even when you are asleep, it's working. Renewing cells, keeping blood pressure steady, growing your hair, growing nails, making new cells as the old ones die, and so on.

Here are some amazing facts about your body:

BEAUTIFUL SKIN

Skin facts
- your entire skin weighs 9lbs
- you get a totally new layer of skin every 40 days
- every square centimetre of skin contains 100 sweat glands

Eye facts
- The orange pigment beta-carotene in carrots, apricots and sweet potatoes is necessary to see in the dark.
- Long lashes need a supply of nutrients, water and a good blood supply from exercise.
- If enough oxygen doesn't reach the eyes, they become bloodshot.

Hair facts
- peak hair growth is from your twenties to forties
- too much vitamin A can cause hair loss
- lack of vitamin A can cause dandruff

If you have been under extreme stress or upset From your break-up, and I assume you have, your body will need a lot of tender loving care.

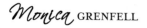
Monica GRENFELL

So let's start with the nutrients you need to feed yourself properly.

1. Protein

Your body might seem much to you as it did a year ago but in that single year, 98% of your old atoms will have been replaced by new atoms which come into your body from the air you breathe, food and water.

The lifespan of cells is 120 days. Each instant of your life, red blood cells, immune cells, hormones and enzymes are being broken down in your body by the sheer wear and tear of living. They are being broken down if you simply lie in bed doing nothing, so imagine how tough life is for your repair system when you're stressed and broken-hearted! They are repaired and maintained with protein. One way of looking at it is to think of your body as a brick wall with protein as the bricks. You can't build a wall with just mortar and sand; you need bricks. The proteins you eat build blood, skin, bone, heart and brain. They also build up and regenerate hormones like insulin, adrenalin and thyroxine which control weight, metabolism and even your sex life. In fact, without proteins, you would fail to thrive, your tissues would leak and you would die.

How much protein you need in one day

Proteins are complex. They are made up of any one of thousands of combinations of just 24 amino acids but eight of these amino acids (called 'essential' amino acids) are the important ones which your body cannot make itself and has to get from food. I am making particular mention of amino acids because they are the most important factors in getting your looks and body looking and feeling

Monica GRENFELL

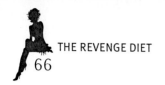
better. Amino acids are your most powerful tools in the process of growing that totally new you!

When you have a stressful time, the body doesn't get enough fuel and in time, this deficit shows. Falling hair, brittle nails, and rough skin are the usual signs, along with poor muscle tone and anaemia. If you don't eat your daily dose of protein over a long period of time, depression, fatigue, infections and skin breakages can result, along with swollen ankles, wrinkles and signs of early ageing.

Sounds good, eh?

2. Carbohydrates

Carbohydrates supply your body with energy. Think of them as petrol in your engine. In recent years, people have identified starchy carbohydrates like bread, rice and pasta, as 'carbs' which they should avoid at all costs. But all vegetable matter is a carbohydrate. In fact, a reliable rule of thumb is to ask yourself if something was once a leaf, seed, grain, fruit or vegetable and if so, it is carbohydrate.

But hang on . . .

Where does milk fit it?

Easy, it comes from grass.

What about yogurt?

Ditto – it comes from milk which comes from grass.

And fruit is carbohydrate?

Absolutely!

Monica GRENFELL

And we need those carbs! Carbs are energy. Yes, all food provides energy, but the beauty of carbs lies in the speed the energy gets into your bloodstream.

But if you're going to lose fat something has to go in your diet and starchy carbohydrates are top foods for the chop. Bread, potatoes and pasta are all nutritious, but they are LESS nutritious, ounce for ounce, than fish, meat, cheese and so on. Bread needs something on it. Pasta merely adds the base and the energy to a meal of meat or vegetables. Bread is the carrier for a toast topping or sandwich filling. So these are the first to go.

Blood sugar levels

People talk about having low blood sugar as if this were an illness or disorder when in fact everybody's blood sugar levels go down as they get hungry and rise quickly when they have eaten a meal.

One of today's problems is eating carbohydrates as if we were still mining coal for a living, using 5,000 calories a day. In fact, we use a fraction of the calories we used to use.

On this diet, you will be eating around 100g carbohydrate a day, which should help use the stocks or energy you already have, and provide enough for each day.

Those carbs will be:
- Milk
- Yogurt
- Fruits
- Vegetables

Monica GRENFELL

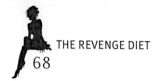
3. Fat

You need around 25g/1oz of fat a day for the body to absorb fat-soluble vitamins. The best way to calculate your 25 g is to read food information labels on bought products.

Omega-3 fatty acids are needed in small amounts, and can be found in:
• A handful of walnuts
• A 100 g/4 oz oily fish such as mackerel
• 2 teaspoonfuls vegetable oil (as in a salad dressing)

Omega-6 fatty acids, found in nuts, seeds and polyunsaturated oils, are needed in similar amounts.

Fats can also be obtained from avocado pears, dairy products and meat.

Remember that eating fatless dishes such as a fatless sponge cake, meringues or boiled rice, can still put on weight if you eat too much of them. None of these foods contains fat, but they still contain calories. Countless good cooks write and tell me they have not eaten a fast-food item in their lives and their entire diet consists of simple, fat-free, home-made meals. So why are they several stones overweight, they ponder?

Well, rice and potatoes are fat-free also, steak and kidney pie is natural and additive-free but the calorie argument prevails: food contains calories, however additive-free, healthy or fatless.

The best fats are monounsaturated or polyunsaturated, and these come from seeds, nuts, fish and some oils. This is fat that stays liquid when cold.

4. Calcium
You need 800mg for adult women aged 18-50, 700mg over 50 and 700mg for men.
(Pregnant and breastfeeding women add 550 mg)

5. Iron
14mg per day
You can usually get this amount from two bowls of fortified cereal or one small steak.

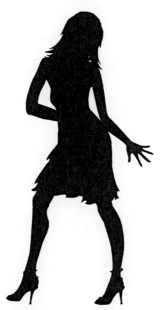

Monica GRENFELL

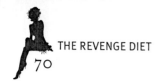

9. Your CORE DIET

The basics of this diet are things most of us have in our storecupboards and fridges – eggs, milk, fruit, yogurt... Nothing fancy or expensive or difficult to find.

Here are the key items:

Milk

Inexpensive, easily available, and a 'complete food'. This means it has all three main nutrients our bodies need; protein, carbohydrate and fat. Skimmed milk is the best as the fat content is low, but you may drink semi-skimmed if you find this more palatable.

Nutritional values
Skimmed:

- 19.4g protein per pint
- 29.2g carbohydrate
- 0.6g fat
- 704mg calcium
- 194 calories

Semi skimmed:
The same as skimmed but with 9.4g fat and 270 calories per pint

Soya:

- 17g protein
- 4.6g carbohydrate
- 11.2g fat
- 188 calories

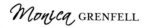

Yogurt

Plain, Fatfree 'bio' yogurt is the ideal snack. A complete food, it is also low-calorie and the ideal accompaniment to fruit and breakfast cereal.

Nutritional values:
Fatfree per 150g pot:
- 5.8g Protein
- 7.2g carbohydrate
- 0.1g fat
- 55 calories

Cheese

Lowfat Cottage cheese is the obvious choice, but all cheese is good. It's the quantity that makes a diet work for you, and as with all meals on this diet, eat small portions.

Nutritional values:
Cottage — small tub:
- 15g protein
- 3.7g carbohydrate
- 1.0g saturated fat
- 87 calories

Cheddar, 30g/1oz.
- 10.2g protein
- Trace carbohydrate
- 8.7g saturated fat
- 120 calories

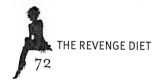
Eggs

Powerhouses of protein, low calorie and very nourishing. Lots of great things happen to your body as a result of eggs. They are good for hair and skin and muscles. In fact, as long as you don't overdo them, you can't go far wrong with eggs!

Nutritional Values
1 large egg:
• 6.3g protein
• trace carbohydrate
• 1.5g saturated fat.
• 80 calories

Oranges

The perfect accompaniment to eggs. Packed with natural carbohydrate, you get energy, sweetness and of course lots of lovely vitamin C when you have pure orange juice. I recommend you only drink orange juice that has actually been squeezed from fresh oranges, and you might want to do this yourself. But a large glass of pure orange juice with an egg meal will fill you for hours.

Nutritional Values
1 large orange:
• 1.8g protein
• 13.6g carbohydrate
• 60 calories

Fish

All fish is good, and we don't forget white fish which is particularly low-calorie.

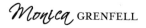

Nutritional Values
Salmon 6oz/150g
- 24.2g protein
- Nil carbohydrate
- 2.5g saturated fat.
- 215 calories

Cod 6oz/150g
- 25.7 protein
- Trace carbohydrate
- 0.4g saturated fat
- 115 calories

Red meat

Red meat really is the best source of iron in the diet as well as being high in protein. In fact, a small fillet steak will supply your entire day's protein and iron requirements.

Nutritional Values

8oz steak
- 48.2g protein
- nil carbohydrate
- 7.4g saturated fat.
- 336 calories

Chicken
- 38.7g protein
- Nil carbohydrate
- 1.2g saturated fat
- 190 calories

Monica GRENFELL

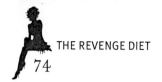
Fruit and vegetables

Fruit and vegetables aren't just there because they are low-calorie and 'good for you'. The body needs fibre to get rid of your waste and most fibre comes from seeds and vegetation. I don't overdo the amount of fruit and veg in this diet, but you will get your 5 portions a day. I also include regular avocado pears. Avocados are amazing fruits with particularly high amounts of vitamins and healthy fats. These help your looks a great deal.

Nuts

Always, always, eat your day's requirement of nuts. Brazil nuts, in particular, contain the anti-oxidant mineral selenium and this is a powerful beauty mineral as well as being good for fighting infections and even cancer. Walnuts and almonds are also amazing and I recommend you have a small palmful each day.

General guidelines

1. Stick to the meals as suggested.
2. Never skip a meal – even if you aren't hungry.
3. Keep to portion sizes.
4. NEVER have second helping.
5. Serve enough food for the meal and never keep leftovers
6. Drink plain water throughout the day.
7. Never have a high protein meal in the evening.

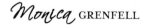

Breakfast
HIGH protein, e.g.
- Eggs
- Milk
- Yogurt

Mid-morning
Yogurt or milk

Lunch
Try and start lunch with either tomato juice or bowl of melon chunks or slice of melon. This takes the edge off the appetite and of course, is nutritious. Lunch should always be a LIGHT meal: this helps you keep a clear head, it keeps blood sugar levels steady and feeds your body and looks. I suggest one of the Main Meal salads if you feel up to the preparation, otherwise you can stick with cheese and fruit, cottage cheese, cold meats or fish and salad.

Mid afternoon
Yogurt or milk

Evening meal
As with lunch, it helps to have a light 'starter' before dinner or a colourful mixed, dressed salad.

Then, for the first six days, dinner should be a simple yet tasty meal of rice with vegetables.

YOU SHOULD NOT EAT
Meat, Fish, Cheese or sauces

Supper
(every night)
- Fresh fruit salad
- Yogurt
- 3 Brazil nuts or 6 almonds

Monica GRENFELL

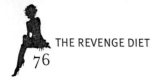
To drink

OK – this is always the party-pooper. Alcohol might be fattening, but its worse crime is in helping you have the 'sod-it' factor. That means you start the evening determined not to lay waste to the buffet like a plague of locusts, but you get tipsy and do it anyway.

So stick to a little red wine – and nothing else! And only at weekends!

Always drink water during the day, especially between meals.

Plus NO diet drinks, NO 'no calorie' flavoured water drinks, NO extra fresh fruit juices

But the good news is you can have tea, coffee, decaf coffee and herbal teas if you wish.

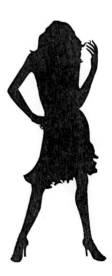

Day 1 – 5

One of the problems of everyday eating is . . .

Too much choice!!

So . . . you're going to love this. For the first five days your meals are nutritionally balanced but very low in calories so you're not piling on more and more calories where you don't need them.

It's also repetitive (but that's good) and steers you away from the pressure of choice. Plus it'll keep you out of the kitchen!

Breakfast

(Ok there's a bit of choice here, but not much!)
Mixed strawberries raspberries and blueberries with sliced mango and apple. Topped with 1 small pot fatfree bio yogurt

or

EGGS AND ORANGE

2 whole eggs and 1 egg white, as either an omelette or scrambled. 250 ml freshly-squeezed orange juice

or

dish of grapefruit segments

or

MONICA'S MUESLI

This is a special recipe based on the original Bircher muesli from around 1900 .

2 tbs oats
½ teacup skimmed milk
1 dsp Fatfree plain yogurt
½ apple, grated
Dsp chopped hazelnuts

Monica GRENFELL

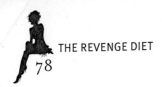
Cover the oats with the milk and leave either overnight or an hour or so . . . Mix the grated apple and hazelnuts (a good idea is to put slices of apple and some whole nuts into a blender and blitz all together) Fold into the yogurt and then fold the yogurt and oats together. This makes a rather sticky, un-crunchy muesli. Serve with a drizzle of honey on top, if desired.

Mid morning
Glass of skimmed or semi-skimmed milk
or
150g pot fatfree bio yogurt (plain)

Lunch
Always start with a small (300ml) glass tomato juice

CHEESE AND FRUIT
Six small cubes of hard cheese, (about the size of dice)
1 segmented apple
12 grapes
3 sticks celery

Mid afternoon
150g pot bio yogurt, as mid-morning

Dinner
180g mixed rice, (brown, wild rice, red rice etc, as you choose) Topped with plenty of grilled, roasted or stir-fry vegetables. Top with a handful of toasted pine nuts Try adding soy sauce or a dessertspoon of half-fat crème fraiche to the vegetables before serving

Supper
Fresh fruit salad
2 dsps of yogurt and 3 Brazil nuts

Monica GRENFELL

Day 6

Now you have more choice, if you wish, with inventive high-protein salad recipes from my suggestions in the recipe section.

If these are too fancy for you DON'T WORRY – You can stay with cheese and fruit or a plain salad but – NO STARCH. Meaning no bread, potatoes pasta or rice.

AT ANY STAGE you may return to the menus for the first week if this suits you.

Breakfast, Mid-morning and Mid-afternoon
As Day 1

Lunch
Tomato juice or melon
Avocado and prawns on salad with vinaigrette dressing
or
Your choice from salad recipes

Mid-afternoon
Yogurt

Dinner
Starter Salad
Pasta with smoked salmon, crème fraiche and dill
or
Jacket potato with winter salad (grated carrot, white and red cabbage, apple, handful sultanas, broken walnuts bound in a very small amount of mayonnaise)

Supper
Mixed fruit salad with 2 dsps fromage frais
3 Brazil nuts or 6 almonds or walnuts

Monica GRENFELL

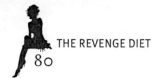
Day 7

Breakfast
As Day 1

Lunch
Cottage cheese and fruit platter
(2 dsp cottage cheese in a scooped-out orange, surrounded by a sliced banana, mango chunks, pineapple, half an apple, sliced and any berries to hand)
or
Sunday lunch (roast meat or poultry with vegetables, no potatoes)
Stewed apple with cinnamon and sultanas, dsp yogurt

Dinner or Tea
Mixed salad
4 avocado and walnut sandwiches with a little walnut oil and lemon dressing (Slice half an avocado, add 4 finely chopped walnuts and mix well. Sandwich in lightly buttered granary bread and add a drizzle of walnut oil and lemon)
or
Salad sandwiches
or
Stir-fry vegetables with rice as first week.

Supper
Mixed exotic fruit salad with mango, pineapple, grapes and kiwi

Day 8

Breakfast
As Day 1

Lunch
Cold chicken breast in Simple Coronation sauce
(dsp mayonnaise, tsp apricot jam, tsp mild curry powder,
mixed well, coating the chicken. Cut into slices or cubes)
Served on shredded lettuce and watercress salad
or
Carrot and celery sticks with 3 tbs houmous or chick pea dip
or
(Eating out) choose steak, grilled chops
or
Fish with plain steamed vegetables
1 apple

Dinner
Mixed salad starter
Pasta with stir-fried vegetables and crème fraiche
or
Baked potato and 4 tbs baked beans
or
Stir-fry vegetables with rice as first week

Supper
Either Fresh fruit salad
or
Stewed apple
Yogurt
3 brazil nuts.

Monica GRENFELL

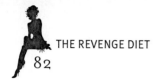

Day 9

Breakfast and Mid-morning
As Day 1

Lunch
Spiced Lamb Salad with Mango dressing*
or
Cheese with apple, celery and grapes
or
(Eating out) choose grilled salmon or white fish with
spinach and carrots (no dessert, but a little cheese and
celery without biscuits is fine if you didn't choose cheese
for lunch itself)

Mid-afternoon
Yogurt

Dinner
Vegetable Curry with salad
or
Half a vegetable pizza with olives, mixed colourful
salad including peppers, grated carrot

Supper
2 pieces of fruit
or
Mixed fruit salad
3 Brazils or 6 almonds or walnuts

*see recipes

Day 10

Breakfast
As Day 1

Lunch
Chicken with Watermelon and Hazelnut Salad with Raspberry vinaigrette*
or
(Very low calorie) Cheese, grapes, celery and apple
or
(Eating out) Plain grilled white fish e.g. sea bass, cod etc, fresh vegetables, no potatoes or bread
Ask for no sauce or butter

Dinner
Pasta with vegetables and crème fraiche
or
Home made pizza Ciabatta slice (half Ciabatta only) with olives, tomatoes, parmesan cheese, capers and goats' cheese, grilled and drizzled with olive oil

Supper
Fromage frais with fruit compote

*see recipes

Monica GRENFELL

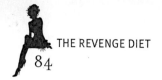
Day 11

Breakfast and Mid-morning
As Day1

Lunch
Tomato juice or melon
2 slices smoked salmon with capers, crème fraiche and salad
or
Your choice from salad recipes
or
Cold chicken or 3 slices ham with 2 sliced tomatoes

Dinner
Mixed salad
Vegetable stir-fry with soy sauce and small jacket
potato
or
Tomatoes on 2 slices toast, scraping of butter

Supper
Fruit salad with fromage frais
Nuts

Day 12

Breakfast and Mid-morning
As Day 1

Lunch
Tomato juice or melon
Tuna Fish salad (without potatoes)
or
(Eating out) Steak and salad
or
Your choice from salad menus

Mid-afternoon
Yogurt

Dinner
Mixed salad
Mushroom and Pine nut risotto
or
Jacket potato and baked beans with salad
or
400ml Lentil soup with 1 slice granary bread

Supper
Fruit, yogurt and nuts

Monica GRENFELL

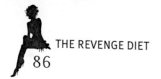
Day 13

Breakfast and Mid-morning
As Day 1

Lunch
Tomato juice or melon
Crab, grapefruit and avocado salad on salad greens
or
Cottage cheese and banana
or
Your choice from salads recipes

Dinner
Mixed salad
1 slice spinach and tomato or asparagus quiche
Green vegetables 2 new potatoes
Carrot or spinach soup with one wholemeal roll
or
Pasta Primavera*

Supper
Poached pears with crème fraiche

Day 14

Breakfast
As Day 1

Lunch
Tomato juice or melon
Avocado and pine nuts salad
or
Sunday lunch (roast meat with all vegetables, no potatoes,
Yorkshire pudding etc)
Baked Apple, fromage frais

Dinner or Tea
Mixed Salad
Small vegetable pizza with colourful mixed salad
or
Salad sandwiches on multigrain bread
or
Avocado and walnut sandwiches on granary bread with
walnut oil

Supper
Fruit, celery and nuts

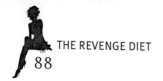

Recipes

CHICKEN HAZELNUT, PEA AND WATERCRESS SALAD

To serve 4

You will need
2 celery stalks, each cut into 4
1 large carrot, quartered
Large handful skinned, toasted hazelnuts
1 tbs lemon juice
3 handfuls of cooked peas
2 bunches watercress
4 tbs olive oil
2 cooked, cold chicken breasts cut into large chunks

Method
Take half the toasted hazelnuts and grind them quickly in a food processor, until still rough. Make a dressing by outing the olive oil in a screw-top jar with the lemon juice and adding the ground hazelnuts. If you like, you can add a thinly slices lemon grass stalk. Give a good shake.

Mix the peas with the watercress and remaining whole hazelnuts and divide between four plates. Sit the chicken pieces on top and drizzle with the dressing.

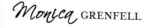 GRENFELL

SALAD OF GRILLED BACON, SOFT-BOILED EGG, BROAD BEANS AND RADISHES, WITH A PEAR DRESSING

To make 2

You will need
2 eggs
300g cooked back bacon
1 pear, cored
6 radishes, sliced thinly.
150g cooked broad beans
2 tbs lemon juice
A handful crunchy lettuce leaves shredded

For the dressing
2 tbs olive oil
1 tbs red wine vinegar
1 tbs soy sauce

Method
Make dressing first – mix the oil, vinegar and soy sauce in a screw top jar and shake well to incorporate. Soft boil the eggs for 4 minutes and cool quickly with shell on, in cold water. Shell the eggs. Heat a dry pan and fry the bacon – you won't need any oil.

Remove from pan and drain on kitchen towel. Dice pears and mix with the radishes, broad beans and lemon juice.

To serve – Toss the crunchy lettuce with the pears and radishes and divide between 2 plates (or out one portion aside to save) Place the bacon on top then rest an egg on top of that, cut in half. Spoon the dressing over and serve.

Monica GRENFELL

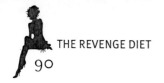
CHICKEN, PRAWN, AVOCADO, ALMOND AND MANGO SALAD

To make 2 portions

You will need
1 avocado
2 chicken breasts, skinless and cooked.
1 mango
Large handful cooked prawns
Handful of whole almonds, toasted
Bunch of watercress
Lettuce leaves
1 tbs lemon juice
1 tbs avocado oil
Handful of bean sprouts

Method

Cut the chicken into chunks and place in large bowl. Cut the avocado in half and remove stone and skin. Cut avocado into chunks and add to the chicken. Peel the mango and slice the flesh away from the centre, cut into chunks. Add the prawns almonds, lettuce and watercress to the chicken and avocado in the bowl.

Make dressing by mixing the lemon juice and avocado oil. Toss the salad in half the dressing, divide between 2 plates (Or save a portion without dressing). Scatter with the beansprouts and drizzle some more dressing round.

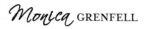

Monica GRENFELL

SCALLOP, ROASTED BUTTERNUT SQUASH, PEANUT, LIME AND CHILI SALAD

To serve 4

you will need
1 large butternut squash
3 tbs ground peanut oil (or any oil like sunflower)
2 tbs spy sauce
20 scallops
Handful of salad greens
Small bunch fresh coriander
Lime wedges to serve

For the dressing
Handful toasted peanuts
1 red chilli roughly chopped
1 clove garlic (optional)
3-4 limes plus tsp grated lime zest
2 tbs brown sugar
2 tsp Thai fish sauce
100ml lime juice

Method

Heat the oven to 180C gas 4. Peel the squash, slit in half, discard seeds. Cut into small chunks, toss in the peanut oil and soy sauce and place in roasting dish with a few tbs hot water. Roast until cooked, about 20 minutes. Leave to cool.

Meanwhile, fry the scallops in a frying-pan with a little oil. Turning a few times. Place the peanuts in a food processor. Tip them into a bowl and add the chilli garlic, lime zest sugar, fish sauce and lime juice. Add the scallops. To the dressing, then add half the peanuts and the coriander and toss everything together.

Monica GRENFELL

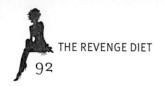
To serve – Divide the squash between 4 plates, top with the greens and then divide the scallops on top of that. Drizzle with the remaining dressing. Scatter the remaining peanuts on top and serve with lime wedges on the side.

COURGETTE, APPLE, HAZELNUT AND ASPARAGUS SALAD

To serve 4

You will need
4 Courgettes
24 asparagus spears, blanched for 2 minutes and refreshed in cold water
2 handfuls toasted hazelnuts
Assorted salad greens
4 eating apples

Dressing
250ml apple juice
6 tbs balsamic vinegar
125ml olive oil

Method
Make the dressing first. Put the apple juice and vinegar in a pan, boil and reduce by 3/4. Leave to cool and then mix in then olive oil

Peel the Courgette into ribbons or slice thinly. Cut the asparagus spears into short lengths. Roughly chop the hazelnuts. Divide the greens between 4 plates. Peel and quarter the apples, thinly slice them and add to the bowl with all the remaining ingredients.

Toss well with the dressing, divide between the plates and drizzle a little more dressing over and around.

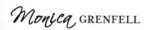

PRAWN OR CRAYFISH, AVOCADO, GINGER AND GRAPEFRUIT SALAD

To serve 2

you will need
Small piece of fresh ginger
1 tbs fresh lime juice
1 tbs caster sugar
2 grapefruits, segmented, or use a tin of pink
grapefruit segments, juice reserved
1 avocado
Handful rocket pr salad leaves
200g prawns or crayfish tails

Dressing
1 tbs avocado oil
1 tbs olive oil
1 tbs balsamic vinegar
Reserved grapefruit juice

Method

Peel and grate or slice the ginger thinly. Mix the ginger with the lime juice and sugar. Segment the fruit or drain the tinned grapefruit. Cut avocados in half and twist out the stone. Cut flesh into large wedges. Make the dressing by mixing all the ingredients and season with black pepper.

To serve – Put the salad leaves and avocado onto 2 plates (or make one serving of this salad and save the rest without dressing, in fridge – will keep for one day) Lay the prawns on top and scatter the grapefruit segments and the ginger. Add the dressing and then mix carefully.

Monica GRENFELL

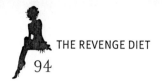

GREEN LENTIL, STILTON AND WALNUT SALAD WITH BROAD BEANS

To serve 4

You will need
250 ml green lentils
100g Stilton cheese
20 whole walnuts
100g cooked broad beans

Dressing
1 tbs sesame seed oil
1 tbs olive oil
1 tbs balsamic vinegar

Method
Mix all ingredients together gently.
Make the dressing by incorporating all the ingredients in a screw top jar and shaking. Divide the salad between 4 plates, allowing the lentils to be a base for the other ingredients.

Pour half the dressing over the salad and mix. Put onto the plates then drizzle the remainder of the dressing over.

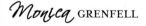

PASTA SALAD WITH AVOCADO DRESSING

To serve 4

You will need
100 g/4 oz pasta shapes
Salt and freshly ground black pepper
50 g/2 oz asparagus, trimmed, tips removed and stalks
cut into 2.5 cm/1 inch pieces
1 courgette, trimmed and sliced
1 large ripe avocado
100 g/4 oz very low-fat fromage frais
½ tbs lemon juice
½ clove garlic, peeled and crushed
½ eating apple
1 tbs chopped fresh coriander

Method

Cook the pasta shapes, according to the packet instructions, adding the asparagus stalk pieces 7 minutes before the end of the cooking time and the courgettes and asparagus tips 2–3 minutes before the end of the cooking time. When the pasta and vegetables are cooked, drain well, and rinse under cold running water, then drain well again. Place in a large bowl.

Cut the avocado in half and remove the stone, then scoop out the flesh from one half and mash in a bowl. Add the fromage frais, lemon juice, garlic, salt and pepper and mix well together. Chop the remaining avocado half into small pieces. Core and chop the apple. Pour the avocado dressing over the pasta and add the chopped avocado and apple. Toss together until mixed, then sprinkle with the coriander. Serve immediately.

Monica GRENFELL

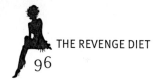
MUSHROOM AND PINE NUT RISOTTO

To serve 2

You will need
200 g/7 oz dry weight risotto rice
30 g/1 oz butter
1 onion, finely chopped
1 clove garlic, crushed
200 g/7 oz mushrooms, sliced
2 tbs toasted pine nuts
2 tps tomato purée
4 tbs half-fat crème fraîche
Salt and freshly ground black pepper
Pinch of nutmeg
Pinch of paprika

Method

Cook the rice according to the packet instructions. Melt the butter in a large frying-pan. Add the onion and garlic and cook over a low heat until transparent. Add the mushrooms. Keep stirring until coated with the butter. Add the rice and stir in the tomato purée, pine nuts and crème fraîche. Add the salt, pepper and nutmeg and cook for a further 2–3 minutes. Sprinkle with paprika and serve immediately.

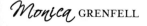 *Monica* GRENFELL

CHICKEN WITH WATERMELON AND HAZELNUT SALAD AND RASPBERRY VINAIGRETTE.

This dish makes plain grilled chicken suddenly sensational. Save time by having raspberry vinaigrette and toasted hazelnuts always in your pantry.

I fillet breast of chicken per person
75g toasted hazelnuts
½ medium seedless watermelon
Bunch torn lambs lettuce
Cup fresh raspberries

Raspberry vinaigrette

50g fresh raspberries
50ml hazelnut oil
25mls raspberry vinegar (a must)

Method

First, process all the vinaigrette ingredients until pureed. Pour through a sieve to get rid of the seeds. To toast hazelnuts, either put them into a hot oven or under grill, without any oil, and keep shaking or put into a dry large frying pan and keep shaking as they gradually turn brown. Take away from heat and leave – (they will keep cooking in their own oil and be extremely hot to touch, so take care.)

Grill the chicken with a spray of oil, until cooked through. Cut the watermelon into chunks. Combine in a bowl with the raspberries/cranberries and lettuce. Slice the chicken thinly or dice, drizzle with the vinaigrette and sprinkle with the nuts. Combine gently with all the other ingredients and serve

Monica GRENFELL

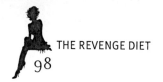
SPICED LAMB SALAD WITH MANGO DRESSING

First get your spices sorted: I recommend making a larger amount and keeping in a screw top jar, to save work next time to make this delicious dish!

2 tbs ground cumin
2 tbs ground coriander
1 tbs ground turmeric
1 tsp hot paprika
2 tsp garlic salt

8oz lamb steak
1 medium red and one yellow capsicum, sliced thinly.
1 onion, sliced thinly
2 medium avocados, sliced thinly.
Lettuce and coriander leaves

Mango dressing

8oz mango and the juice of 2 limes blended

Method

Simply mix the spices in a screw-top jar and shake.

Place the lamb in a bowl with as much of the spice mix as you would like to use, for personal preference. Keep the rest for another time. Roll until all sides are covered, leave for 30 minutes up to overnight. Cook the lamb in shallow oil until browned all over and to the pinkness you prefer. Rest 5 minutes then slice thinly. Mix the lamb with the red, green or yellow peppers, avocado, lettuce, onion and coriander, drizzle with dressing and serve.

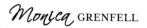

Monica GRENFELL

LINGUINI IN CREAMY WATERCRESS SAUCE

To serves 2

You will need
I tablespoon vegetable oil
I medium onion, finely chopped
I clove garlic, crushed (optional)
125 ml/4 fl oz dry white wine
125 ml/4 fl oz fish stock
I tsp cornflour
150 ml/5 fl oz single cream
2 bunches firmly packed watercress, trimmed
225 g/8 oz linguini
Salt and freshly ground black pepper

Method

Heat the oil in a large pan. Add the onion and garlic and cook over a low heat until soft. Add the wine and stock and boil until reduced by one third, stirring continuously. Blend the cornflour with a little of the cream. Add with the remaining cream to the pan and keep stirring until the mixture thickens. Remove from the heat and add the watercress. You can blend the sauce in a food processor if you prefer it smooth.

Meanwhile, cook the linguini according to the packet instructions and add to the sauce in the pan. Season to taste with salt and pepper. Serve immediately.

Monica GRENFELL

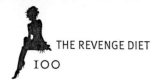
PASTA PRIMAVERA

To serve 1

You will need
100 g/4 oz fresh pasta spirals or quills
2 tbs olive oil
Handful mixed mangetout, baby sweetcorn, sugar-snap
peas, carrot sticks, red and green peppers, beansprouts
I tsp pesto sauce
2 tsp crème fraîche
Salt and freshly ground black pepper

Method
Cook the pasta according to the packet instructions. Drain and keep warm. Heat the oil in a deep frying-pan or wok, and add the mixed vegetables. Toss over a high heat for 1 minute. Add the pasta and the pesto sauce. Turn for 30 seconds. Remove from the heat, add the crème fraîche, season to taste with salt and pepper and serve immediately.

For more delicious recipes visit www.monicagrenfell.co.uk and follow the link to *The Revenge Diet*.

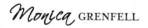 GRENFELL

... a word about **EXERCISE**

It's easy to let yourself go when you feel depressed and hopeless. But you must never let any situation get so bad that it takes over your body as well as your mind.

Exercise will make things better. Fresh air will invigorate you and if you can get breathless, panting, sweaty perhaps ... the extra blood flow to your skin is FABULOUS for your complexion.

In fact ...

Sitting around and getting sluggish gives you spots, clogs the pores and will produce those white, hard spots under your eyes, on your eyelids and cheeks that are so hard to get rid of, and which say ...

I'm a mess! SO ...

Get going on this programme – no excuses – and see how much better you look and feel.

DAY 1	40–60 MINUTES CARDIO	E.g. Cycling, swmming, aerobics class
DAY 2	20 MINUTES UPPER BODY TONING	Using weights for shoulders, arms, chest and back
DAY 3	40–60 MINUTES CARDIO	As Day 1
DAY 4	REST DAY	
DAY 5	CARDIO AS DAY 1	As Day 1
DAY 6	20 MINUTES TONING, 30 MINUTES YOGA, PILATES OR STRETCH	Inner and outer thighs, backs of thighs. Use DVD or stretch class
DAY 7	60 MINUTES PLUS GENERAL WALKING OR LIGHT EXECISE	Try to go for endurance walk of 2–3 hours or gardening, car washing etc.

Find out much more on www.monicagrenfell.co.uk

Monica GRENFELL

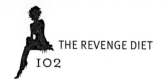

10. Your QUESTIONS answered

Q. This diet really suited me. Is it OK to stay on it for the long term?

A. Yes it is. This diet has all you need in terms of nutrition, though I do recommend nursing mothers, pregnant women and growing teens take an iron supplement. My recommendation would be one called SPATONE which is totally natural, iron-rich water from the mountains of Snowdonia, which you add to orange juice. In fact, I recommend all women take this supplement – it is the only one I take regularly (www.spatone.co.uk).

The diet is high in protein, calcium, vitamins and minerals and low in fat and calories. If you are maintaining weight you can simply increase portion sizes but never, ever add sweet, starchy or 'junk' items like biscuits and cakes – well, not more than once a week anyway!

Q. I often eat out in the evening or go to friends and I might fancy a steak or other high protein item. I see that we shouldn't have too much protein in the evening as it can interfere with digestion. What do you suggest – should I do my own thing or eat what I am given?

A. I have one golden rule in these circumstances –

never let lean make you mean.

Monica GRENFELL

If someone has gone to the trouble of making you something, get on and eat it and never complain, discuss your intolerances or bring your diet to everyone's attention! This is simply bad manners.

As long as you are eating good, pure food, it won't matter at all if you have meat or chicken or fish – nothing terrible is going to happen to you. The worst thing will be indigestion or a feeling of fullness. But it won't affect your weight loss.

Q. There are a lot of eggs on this programme. I like eggs but isn't there a cholesterol problem?

A. No, because dietary cholesterol tends not to raise total cholesterol and you don't take in cholesterol from your food to such a great extent. High cholesterol is usually caused by the body's inability to deal with it, such as an impaired liver function, rather than eating it in food.

The eggs in this diet are mostly egg whites with only the odd whole egg with yolk. Egg whites are pure protein, exceptionally low-calorie at just ten calories each, and they have no cholesterol.

Q. I really don't like dairy food, which tends to cause wheezing problems – I am probably slightly intolerant. Can I substitute soya products?

A. Of course you can – they are nutritious and some people simply prefer the taste. However, I am recommending a diet that gets best results and as you have read, dairy calcium is particularly implicated in fat loss. If you don't have dairy this might influence the results, but I don't want you to eat anything you really can't face, so do go ahead and enjoy your soya products. It's the natural state of food that counts in the long run.

Monica GRENFELL

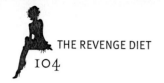
Q. Why do you say we must eat a salad before our main meal?

A. Well, apart from the fact that it's good for you, it takes the edge off the appetite and this might stop you piling into your main course, ravenous, and eating slightly more than you should. Salad is vegetation, obviously, and the body really needs plenty of leaves and seeds and fruits to add fibre to the diet, which in turn cleanses the system nicely. Diets without much fibre do leave you extremely constipated if you regularly avoid fruit and vegetables.

Q. Can I miss a meal if I want to lose more weight?

A. Never miss a meal. Your body wants and needs routine so it can get into a rhythm. You might want to lose more weight but actually, skipping meals doesn't really work. You only save a few calories anyway. It's important not to starve your body of nutrients which it needs for that all-important beauty! Far better to eat smaller portions.

Q. I'm really feeling very low and panicky since my split. I can't eat much at all. What do you suggest?

A. Start by drinking milk regularly during the day and having some fruit. This way, you get protein carbohydrate and fat, with fibre thrown in so your body doesn't get constipated and sluggish.
Milk is a great, complete food. If this is tricky, try yogurt. But never ever try and exist on fruit – it has hardly any protein and will do you no good at all in the long run.

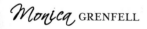 *Monica* GRENFELL

Q. I'm still struggling with the concept of eating a larger meal in the evening. Why won't this make me fat?

A. Because it doesn't! I don't know where this myth started, but plenty of people, like actors, have to eat a meal as late as midnight and they aren't all fat! It's what you eat that counts, and meat or chicken or fish aren't a good idea. Jacket potatoes and pasta, for example, or something on toast, will always digest more easily as long as you allow an hour or so before going to bed afterwards.

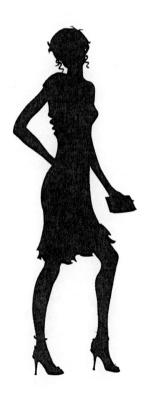

Monica GRENFELL

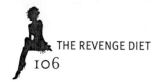

And finally ...

He comes back, he says you're his 'shining star' and you have this great connection.

He wants to see you again.

You're over the moon!! Right??

Then he hits you with it: he's seeing someone else. He wants to see YOU, too, and anything's better than nothing, you tell yourself.

Well you know something?

HE'S NOT INTERESTED IN COMMITMENT

Of Course he wants to see you.

But why would a man have the affections and attention of one woman if he can have two?

This is an essential truth most women just don't get. They say a man is 'having his cake and eating it' and plotting some secret agenda. But a man has no such thoughts. Put it this way – do you have children? If so, you'll know its ludicrous when someone asks if you prefer one child over another. Your kids are different, but you love them equally. You don't think you're 'having you cake and eating it' just because you have the love of all your children.

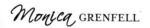
Monica GRENFELL

And it's like this with men. They don't over-analyse but simply get on with the business of fitting as many women into their lives as they can. And loving it!!

OK I know all men aren't like this, so if your husband or loyal boyfriend is reading this and getting furious, apologise from me.

But we're talking now about those who DO mess up your head and if his truth is that he wants to be with you, or not be with you, you have to respect that.

But women do it all the time.

The guy will be sending all kinds of subtle signs that he's not "available" or interested in something "serious", but the woman ignores them and thinks of the fact that he likes being with her.

Wrong!

The first thing a woman does in this situation is try and fix things and convince him she's the one. But by doing this you become far less attractive to him.

This doesn't mean you don't have great times together.

But sometimes this turns into some sort of pressure and your man associates seeing you with feeling less than good – especially if he knows you're going to be asking all sorts of questions or getting 'deep' each time you meet.

So back off.

Monica GRENFELL

- Get back to the things that you enjoy, the places you like to go and avoid places or things you used to do or see with your ex.
- Spend some time with your friends and give yourself some space.
- The less you talk about your ex and this situation the better off you'll be.

And in any case . . .

- Throw away al the CD's you used to play in your car on the way to and from seeing him – they might not be 'your song' but you'll associate them with the journey to his place, whatever. Chuck them out anyway – throw them in a public bin or if you're worried about the waste of money, pack them up and ask a friend to put them in her loft.
- Go through your clothes and do the same
- Delete all the old emails. Again, if you can't bear to do this, (and I've known people who got back together and wished they'd kept the messages and letters) parcel them up or print out and package up, and take them somewhere you can't get at them easily, like a friend's house. One friend took out a safety deposit box! Whatever works for you, do it, but get these things to places where you can't pore over them for hours breaking your heart ten times over.
- Tell yourself that you're a winner, not a loser. Don't flog dead horses. Sometimes, giving in and accepting the reality of a situation can feel like the ultimate failure; like he has won. But he hasn't because you have accepted that winners simply back off and move to the next fun thing. Tell yourself that he has ceased to be fun and you're not interested any more.

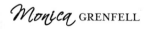

Monica GRENFELL

And now, maybe, if you step back and stop chasing him and trying to convince him you're the one for him, an amazing thing will happen:

- He won't understand where you are and what to do in that space you used to inhabit.
- Which will first get him thinking about you and then wondering why you aren't acting the way you used to.
- And if you can do this, I guarantee he'll come calling wondering about you and . . .

He'll start fancying you all over again

Good luck!!

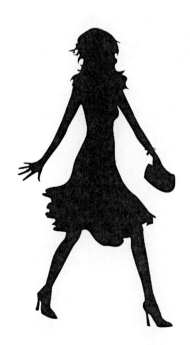

Monica GRENFELL

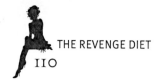
AFTERWORD

I promised I'd tell you what happened when I met the man who broke my heart 23 years ago. The only problem is, I told him about this book, so he'll be reading this. But in fact, it was all good.

We were both clearly older but once we'd got over the fact of being more mature in outlook, we were remarkably the same. His tight, sexy jeans had given way to loose, rather ageing trousers, and I daresay my apparel was no better. Fortunately we'd both kept our shapes. Once he got talking, he was the same 37 year old man I'd known and been passionate about all those years ago and we chatted incessantly. There I was, drinking wine easily with the man who shattered my heart all those years ago. In fact, it did my heart good. He'd just turned 60 but you wouldn't believe it.

He still has a mistress. It turned out he'd been a serial Bad Boy ever since I last saw him, despite being a devoted husband, father and grandfather. But his experience of women was invaluable and as I had problems of my own, he soon became a sounding board, mentor and adviser. Do I fancy him now? No, and he doesn't fancy me. . . If I'd known half the story of our affair from his perspective I wouldn't have stayed with him back then. For a start, he hadn't been as keen on me as I believed. I'd been a convenient weekly diversion and little more. . . "Did you love me?" he asked me.
"Yes"
There was a pause
"And did I say I loved you?"

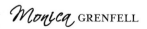
Monica GRENFELL

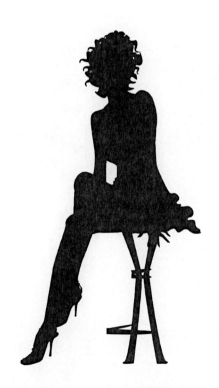

Monica GRENFELL

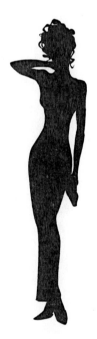

Monica GRENFELL